NUTRITION FOR GASTRIC BAND WEARERS

A Practical Handbook

By

Nicola M. Pearson Bsc (Hons), Dip ION, MBANT, CNHC

and Claudia Williamson Dip ION, MBANT, CNHC

DEDICATION

To my friend Nancy - without you I would never have written this book.

CW

To everyone having difficulties managing their weight. May this book help you in a practical and positive way on your journey.

NP

ACKNOWLEDGEMENTS

We would like to say a big thank you to our friends, colleagues and patients for proof-reading, peer-reviewing and most importantly critiquing the manuscript.

Irene, thank you for reading every version of the book with such enthusiasm, it's done now, you can relax!

Nicola, for your constant positivity and enthusiasm, and for keeping me inspired and motivated, I thank you.

CW

Claudia, thank you for your humour and generous doses of straight talking. You're a wonderful person to work with.

NP

Disclaimer

We are not responsible for your health.

We are not doctors, we are nutritional therapists who want to try and get information about the nutritional implications of being obese and/or having a band to as many people as possible, in an accessible format. We have set out with our best intentions but cannot assume the responsibility of treating you, nor what happens to you if you take this advice. It is not our intention to diagnose, treat, cure or prevent any disease. We just want to share information.

We have had the book peer reviewed by a number of colleagues, gastric band wearers, and bariatric support staff. We take full responsibility for the information within this book, however, we are well aware research is moving at a phenomenal rate and we may therefore have omitted information you feel is important. We welcome all feedback and amendments will be made in future editions, where appropriate.

This area of work and research is changing rapidly and we encourage band wearers to keep in touch with their health team and support group, and for health professionals to use this information in conjunction with their best clinical judgment.

This handbook aims to provide general nutritional advice. It is not a substitute for professional health advice. Always consult an appropriate health professional about your medical problems and keep them informed of any changes.

Choosing a Nutritional Therapy Practitioner

Training:

It is important to choose a qualified Registered Nutritional Therapist who has undertaken all the necessary training to understand the theory and practice of nutritional therapy. For more information follow the link:

www.cnhcregister.org.uk/newsearch/index.cfm

Voluntary Regulation:

By choosing Nutritional Therapists registered with the CNHC you can be confident that they are properly trained, qualified and insured.

Professional Association:

By choosing a Registered Nutritional Therapist who is a member of BANT you can be confident that they follow the strict CNHC Code of Conduct, Performance and Ethics and the BANT Professional Practice Handbook, have professional indemnity insurance for clinical practice and also meet the membership entry criteria found at this link:

www.bant.org.uk/nutritional-therapy-careers/join-bant/apply-formembership/full-membership/

CONTENTS

Chapter 3. Considerations

Chapter 4. Fertility, Preconception and Pregnancy

Chapter 5. Food & Drink

Chapter 6. Nutrients

Chapter 7. Supplements

Chapter 8. Recipes

Chapter 9. Checklists

Chapter 10. Moving Forward

Preface

The overweight are just as malnourished as the starving.

Catherine Bertini, 2006

The need for this book:

The National Institute for Health and Care Excellence (NICE) issued updated recommendations in November 2014, that in order to tackle the type 2 diabetes epidemic the NHS should offer bariatric surgery to thousands more people each year. Guidelines included recent-onset type 2 diabetics with a BMI of 35 or over should be assessed for bariatric surgery, and that weight-loss surgery is beneficial for people who have poorly controlled recent-onset type 2 diabetes with a BMI of 30-34.9 or lower for people of Asian, African, Caribbean and other minority ethnic groups.

A quarter of the UK population is now obese and one in 20 people in the UK has type 2 diabetes. Although the most common types of bariatric surgery performed in the UK last year were gastric bypass and sleeve gastrectomy, these updated guidelines will have a significant impact on the number of gastric band wearers in the UK.

Pregnancy after bariatric surgery is safer than pregnancy in morbidly obese women. Women who have had bariatric surgery generally tolerate pregnancy well. However, there are risks involved and patients must be well informed. Optimal education should be encouraged in these individuals so that they can make well informed decisions about planning pregnancy after their surgery.

Jason Waugh, (2013) Editor-in-Chief, The Obstetrician & Gynaecologist

Introduction

> *Change will not come if we wait for some other person, or if we wait for some other time. We are the ones we've been waiting for. We are the change that we seek.*
>
> Barack Obama, 2008

This book has been written because we discovered a mutual interest in helping people who are overweight, obese or have been fitted with gastric bands. We felt there was a real need for collective, accurate information that was easily accessible for people thinking about getting a band, those with one, and those considering having theirs removed.

When we started (in 2011) there were vast variations between advice and support around the world for gastric band patients, and we wanted to collect clinical experiences and science to support individuals, giving them the knowledge they needed to make their own future health choices. In the four years we have been writing this book, the differences we used to see are now far less. Health professionals are working collectively to share information and best practice, and the scientific community are pulling information together at a great speed. We look forward to the day when guidelines within scientific literature are being followed in clinical practice and people who are considering bands or wearing bands feel empowered with accurate knowledge about how to look after their longer-term health and happiness.

This book has been written for gastric band wearers, those considering having one fitted, or one removed. All the recommendations suggested are backed up with evidence so that you know we are not making up faddy ideas, and also so the book meets the needs of health professionals that are working with gastric band patients. We have tried our hardest not to get bogged down in scientific detail and hope that all of our readers, whatever stage you are at, and whoever you are, manage to find something useful within this book.

Our aim is to inspire gastric band wearers to achieve good (or even great) health and vitality through food – it's not just a question of what you *can* eat but what would be *best* for you to eat – for your long-term health. Stomach capacity is limited so every mouthful needs to be nourishing...

Within this book we start by introducing the band and then discussing what health is and what it means to you. We have then dedicated a section to what else to consider if you are still not achieving your weight-loss goals. This section contains questionnaires under a number of the topics we cover. Next we take a closer look at pre-conception to pregnancy and beyond. The rest of the book focuses on eating and nutrients, foods to include and avoid, and a short section on drinks. We've included "how to eat" with sample weekly menu plans for each phase on your weight-loss journey. The nutrient section covers a range of nutrients and foods commonly deficient in gastric band wearers or in people who are obese. The data is still really limited here so we've tried our hardest to find everything we could. This section is intended to help you determine which nutrient deficiencies may be underlying your inability to lose sufficient weight. In chapter seven, we have included over 45 easy, delicious recipes, full of natural whole foods that are ideal for the gastric band wearer or obese patient to help achieve optimum nutrition. Each chapter is summarised to help pinpoint the key areas from each section that matter to you, and help you identify the changes you feel comfortable to make.

3

Thin or Fat Advice?

Ken Clare from www.wlsinfo.org.uk gave a wonderful presentation on his personal story. He explained that most of the people he works with don't want to take advice from a 'thin' person, they want 'fat' specialists. He continued to say that this was madness, if you have cancer, you don't expect your consultant to also have cancer, so why would you expect this from someone who can help with weight-loss or maintenance?

Neither of us have had bariatric surgery but we have spent years learning about foods, nutrients, excess weight, bariatric surgery, and working with people of all ages and backgrounds, so hopefully you will keep on reading.

Your band is personal.

Your band is totally personal, and therefore no one else can tell you exactly what, or how much, to eat. We don't know the exact size of your pouch or the tightness of your band, nor how it feels for you on each given day. The band is also affected by your emotions, which is why some days you will be able to eat some things that on other days you can't. The band's behaviour can also be affected by other factors such as flying and altitude. Everybody is different and you are the expert on your body and your band. We hope to inspire you to feel and experience that every mouthful really can matter.

Wherever possible we have included information and recommendations from international obesity guidelines. A number of abbreviations are used which include:

- **AACE** = American Association of Clinical Endocrinologists
- **TOS** = The Obesity Society
- **ASMBS** = American Society for Metabolic and Bariatric Surgery
- **BOMSS** = British Obesity and Metabolic Surgery Society

Chapter 1

Gastric Banding - An Overview

> *Go where you are celebrated — not tolerated. If they can't see the real value of you, it's time for a new start.*
>
> Unknown

1.1 What is a gastric band?

A gastric band is a restrictive device that is placed around the upper part of the stomach. The band creates a small pouch at the upper part of the stomach that will hold about 1oz of food immediately after surgery, progressing to 3oz/85ml food for each meal after 3-4 weeks. The pouch is around 1/6 of the size of the full stomach and fills rapidly with food as the band restricts the movement of food to the lower stomach. The idea is that as the upper part of the stomach is filled, the brain receives a message that the entire stomach is full and this sensation helps the person to be hungry less often, to feel full more quickly and for a longer period of time, and to eat smaller portions. The reality is that some patients are always hungry.

The non-adjustable gastric band was the first used at the end of the seventies. In 1986, an adjustable band was introduced which lowered complication rates and improved weight-loss. The internal diameter of the adjustable band can be tightened by inflation of a balloon. As weight is lost saline solution can be injected into a small access point, the injection port, which is placed just under the skin. When fluid is added the band will tighten, further restricting the passage between the upper and lower parts of the stomach, thereby reducing the flow of food. Inflation of the balloon usually begins 6 weeks after surgery and the patient should be seen every 3 months for the first 18 months.

Adjustable Gastric Band Procedure

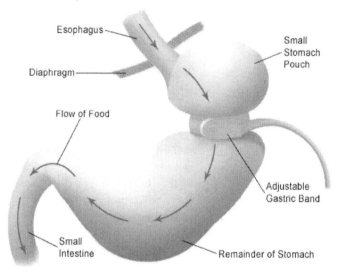

Source: www.hypnotic weightloss.com.au

1.2 Who can have a gastric band?

Gastric band surgery is recommended for people who have a:

✓ Body Mass Index (BMI) ≥ 40

✓ BMI ≥ 35 with two other co-morbid conditions such as hypertension, diabetes or hyperlipidemia

✓ BMI of 30-34.9 in poorly controlled recent-onset type 2 diabetics or lower for ethnic minorities

✓ Exhibited a failure of dietary or weight-loss drug therapy for more than one year

✓ History of obesity (generally 5 years+)

✓ Good understanding of the risks and benefits of the procedure

✓ Willingness to comply with the considerable lifelong dietary restrictions that are required for long term success

✓ Willing to accept the operative risk

Most gastric band patients lose 1 to 2 pounds per week repeatedly, representing about 49 to 99 pounds for the first year.

Banding has satisfactory and safe weight-loss in 80% of patients, not the other 20%.

1.3 The benefits of a band compared with other types of weight-loss surgery

- Lower mortality rate (1 in 2000 compared to 1 in 250 for gastric bypass surgery)
- No stapling or cutting of the stomach
- Fully reversible if required
- Quick recovery rate and short hospital stay
- Easily adjustable without further surgery
- Fewer life threatening complications

1.4 The risks of having a gastric band

- Infections
- Internal bleeding
- Ulcers
- Gastritis
- Blood clots
- Chest pain
- Purpose can be defeated if patient chooses to eat high-caloric liquid diet

1.5 The side effects of having a gastric band

- Vomiting – not considered a complication in the first few months of placement but if beyond 9 months of surgery, positioning of band and dietary habits must be reviewed
- Discomfort

- Inability to ingest some solid foods if incorrectly placed or adjusted
- Constipation
- Hair loss during first 6 months after surgery due to relative starvation
- Infection in the abdomen

1.6 Complications of having a gastric band

- Broken band with subsequent immediate weight gain

- Band slippage is the most frequent late complication, leading to poor weight-loss and severe reflux and heartburn or total inability to eat. If not diagnosed early, can eventually lead to strangulation of the stomach and gastric necrosis

- Band migration – the balloon or band migrates through the stomach wall into the stomach lumen (about 3%) – usually 18-24 months after surgery

- Pouch dilatation – if patient eats too much, satiety is diminished leading to progressive dilatation

- Port (access point) problems –

  - Dislocation of the port (it may move around or turn upside down in which case it can't be injected)

  - Perforation of the connecting tube close to the port (when injecting the saline, especially if patient has extra fat over the chest), resulting in loss of fluid, widening of opening and subsequent weight gain

  - Infection of the port system

1.7 Pre-operation Diet

Your surgeon may ask you to follow a strict diet for two weeks immediately before your surgery. This diet is to help shrink the liver so the surgeon can operate more easily and safely. It is important to follow the diet for the full two weeks before your operation – do not be tempted to have a special meal before surgery as this will reverse the liver-reducing effects of the diet. The recommended diet would be low fat with moderate carbohydrate, and as food is limited it is advisable to take a multivitamin and mineral tablet during this period as well as after surgery.

Protein allowance (2 portions a day) – choose from:

- 2 medium eggs – poached, boiled, scrambled (not fried)
- 100g/4oz sliced ham, chicken or turkey
- Small breast (100g/4oz) of chicken – without skin
- 4 rashers grilled back bacon
- 2 grilled sausages
- 100g/4oz cooked fish – any type
- 100g/4oz very lean cooked meat (with fat cut off)
- 100g4oz tofu
- 100g/4oz low fat cottage cheese
- 150g/1 small pot low fat plain yogurt
- 4 tablespoons cooked lentils, beans (i.e. low sugar baked beans, kidney beans etc)
- 100g/4oz low fat hummus
- 2 tablespoons raw nuts (not roasted and salted)

Starchy carbohydrate allowance (3 portions a day) – choose from:

- 1 slice of wholemeal bread or toast
- ½ wholemeal pitta
- ½ wholemeal bagel
- 3 tablespoons branflakes or oats
- 1½ Weetabix
- 2 oat cakes
- 3 new potatoes (skin on)
- 2 tablespoons cooked rice (preferably brown or basmati)
- 3 tablespoons cooked wholemeal pasta

Vegetable allowance (5 portions a day):

Aim for a wide variety of raw and cooked vegetables and salads each day – e.g. beetroot, broccoli, cabbage, cauliflower, celery, courgette, cucumber, fennel, leeks, lettuce, mushrooms, peppers, radish, spinach, spring onions, tomatoes (tinned and fresh), watercress. If using a salad dressing, choose a low fat option.

- 3 heaped tablespoons cooked vegetables
- 1 cereal bowl sized salad/raw vegetables

Fruit allowance (2 portions a day):

- 1 medium sized fruit such as apple, pear, orange or banana
- 2 small fruit e.g. plums, satsumas, apricots
- 150g/5oz berries – strawberries, raspberries, blueberries

- 1 handful grapes
- 3 tablespoons stewed or tinned fruit (no added sugar)

Condiments/spices – any can be used to add flavour

- Curry powder
- Fish sauce
- Herbs – fresh or dried
- Lemon/lime juice
- Mustard
- Pepper
- Salt
- Soy sauce
- Spices
- Stock cubes
- Thai curry paste
- Vanilla essence
- Vinegar
- Worcester sauce
- Yeast extract

Throughout the day:

- 200ml skimmed or semi-skimmed milk for drinks/cereal.
- Spread your food and drinks throughout the day – don't save everything for one big meal.
- Drink at least 2 litres of hydrating fluid every day – more in hot weather – this includes water, herbal teas, coconut water.
- Drink regularly throughout the day. It's the best way to keep hydrated and is good practice for after your surgery.

- Avoid alcohol.
- Stay busy and active.

Tips for success:

- Planning! – Plan your meals and snacks in advance.
- Eat at regular intervals – your daily plan should include 3 meals and 2 snacks.
- If you find this diet too hard, another option would be using protein shakes and soups – if you feel this would be easier for you.

Diabetics:

If you have diabetes controlled by medication, this will need to be adjusted during the pre-operative diet. As your food intake is reduced, you may need to reduce your medication so check your blood sugar levels regularly. Speak to your GP or practice nurse as they will be able to offer advice on how best to control your diabetes during this time.

1.8 Frequently Asked Questions

If you have any problems with your band we recommend you seek immediate advice from your bariatric team. We have included some of our most commonly asked questions, however, this is not provided as a substitute for medical advice.

What do I do, if I get food stuck in my band?

We recommend that you firstly drink some water and see if that dislodges it. If not, then a small glass of sparkling water may help. Remember which foods cause discomfort and try to avoid them in future. And ensure you are chewing each mouthful really well. If the sparkling water does not resolve the problem, band obstruction is a medical emergency, contact your bariatric team urgently.

I hate fruit and vegetables.

Don't worry you are not alone; we commonly hear this from patients when we first start working together. Firstly go slowly, try one or two new items a week. Or choose one item and try it steamed, or baked and see how the taste differs. There are many varieties of foods, for example some people like crunchy pears and others like juicy ones. You'll be amazed at how your taste buds change as you keep persevering and as you move away from foods high in additives and flavourings.

I'm hungry all the time.

The band has been placed to help reduce your feelings of hunger. As you get used to the smaller portions you may feel hungry out of habit. If this is not the case please speak to your bariatric team.

Are you drinking plenty of hydrating fluids?

Are you having adequate protein with each meal?

Protein helps keep you feeling fuller for longer, gastric band wearers commonly underestimate how much protein they are eating. This may help.

I'm thirsty and feel dehydrated all the time.

Ensure you are sipping water frequently, and focus on foods from the high-water content fruit and vegetable list we have provided in chapter 5.

Help, I'm constipated.

Check that you are drinking enough. And make sure you have adequate fruits, vegetables and pulses in your diet.

Some people find mixing ground flaxseed (or Psyllium husk or ground chia seed) with prune juice and leaving it until it turns mousse like, then eating with a spoon may help. If the problem persists please get support from a health practitioner.

My hormones feel as if they are all over the place.

This can happen after sudden weight-loss and is perfectly normal. Sex drive and menstrual patterns quite frequently change. Let your body have a chance to get used to your new weight and things should settle down again. If not and you are concerned please seek further support. Remember you may need to adjust your contraception while your body and hormones change.

Can't I just have half a sandwich instead of the two I'd have before?

Yes, but… it's not just about having smaller portions, it's about the quality of food you are having. So of course initially go for smaller portions if that is what you are comfortable with, but your eating habits need to change, and the sooner they do the better.

How many pints/glasses of wine can I drink?

Sensibly, it's probably best to tell yourself you no longer drink. We all know what happens after one glass of wine/pint — it's so easy to get another, and then forget what you're doing!

But we live in the real world and know if you are a drinker, you're probably going to drink anyway. On that premise, stick to one glass of wine a week, or one pint (which you may need to have as two slow halves). Then stop.

What about my family – what are they going to eat?

Once you have passed phase 2, you and your family can eat exactly the same food. This is an ideal time for you all to eat more healthily and many families report that working together made the changes so much easier. We recommend working through a weekly menu plan together so everyone has dishes they like. Once you've done this for a few weeks you then have a stockpile of favourites.

Summary:

✓ Gastric bands restrict the amount and movement of food into the stomach

✓ Gastric banding is a reversible procedure

✓ Banding has satisfactory and safe weight-loss in 80% of patients, not the other 20%

✓ Consider and evaluate the benefits, risks, side effects and complications

✓ You may need to follow a strict pre-surgery diet

✓ Frequently Asked Questions

Chapter 2

Health, Fat & Implications of Wearing a Band

> *My body is precious and not separate from my soul.*
>
> SARK

2.1 What is Health?

The World Health Organisation (WHO) says health is "a *state of complete physical, mental, and social well-being and not merely the absence of disease or infirmity*". This statement has been criticised for over 60 years but no one has yet agreed upon a better definition.

2.2 Health Triangle

Let's take a quick look at the "health triangle" which suggests that maintenance and promotion of health is achieved through different combinations of physical, mental, and social well-being (Georgia University, 1998; Nutter, 2003).

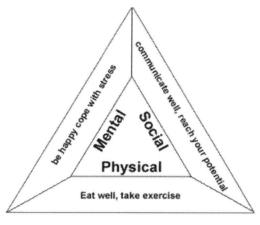

Source: Nutter, 2003

Physical health: is about your body and its ability to function. Nutrition, exercise, sleep, alcohol, smoking, drugs and weight management affect your physical health.

Mental health: is about how we cope with life, how we think and feel about life, and situations that we find ourselves in. This may also include mental health issues such as depression or anxiety. Learning new skills, stress management, meditation and other cognitive studies have all been shown to help.

Social wellbeing: is about you, your family and friends. Are you encouraging, loving and do you feel safe? The community is also important, and may include such things as disease prevention and promoting public health.

What does health mean to you?

> *Challenges are what make life interesting and overcoming them is what makes life meaningful.*
>
> Joshua J. Marine

2.3 Self Management

The Alameda County Study (1982), looked at health habits of 6,298 adults. The outcomes showed that people CAN improve their health via:

- Regular physical exercise
- Sleeping 7-8 hours a night
- Maintaining a healthy body weight
- Limiting alcohol use
- Avoiding smoking (Wingard et al., 1982)

The ability to adapt and to self manage are core components of human health (Huber et al., 2011). So this means your life and your health are in your hands.

> *Lifestyle change is the cornerstone of weight management.*
>
> Freedhoff & Sharma, 2010

2.4 *What is fat doing anyway?*

> *No one wakes up in the morning and says, 'I want to gain
> 150 pounds and I will start right now!'*
>
> Tricia Cunningham

Let's talk a little about fat cells. There are three commonly known fat cells although this area is changing rapidly and probably more are going to be found.

1) Brown cells, which burn up energy, contain iron-rich mitochondria (known also as the 'powerhouse' of cells). Higher numbers of brown fat cells are found in babies (around 5% of total body weight) and decline as we age (Gesta et al., 2007). Brown fat tissue can increase due to environmental changes such as exercise (Matteis et al., 2013) or being in a cold environment (Lee et al., 2014). A number of other factors are also involved in browning white fat and these include vitamin A, the thyroid, liver, muscles, heart, and the immune system (Villarroya & Vidal-Puig, 2013).

2) White cells are made up of a multitude of additional components that include hormones, inflammatory markers, and a number of other chemical compounds. White fat is recognised as an active organ that participates in hormonal and inflammatory processes (Gnacinska et al., 2009; Wozniak et al., 2009).

3) A third kind of fat cell has recently been discovered that is neither white nor brown (Canon & Nedergard, 2012). It's been termed 'beige' or 'brite' adipose tissue (Lanthier & Leclerq, 2014; Pierce et al., 2014). Scientists are currently investigating its role within the body.

Fat generally gets bad press, not only due to the cosmetic and psychological issues of having excess weight, but also because of the association with metabolic disease. However, healthy fat cells have very important properties; these include protecting sensitive areas in the body such as the brain and eyes, cushioning body parts including the heel and toe pads, and for sexual selection, such as the female buttocks. Fat cells key biological functions though are not just to make a beautiful bottom, but play a key role in reproduction via hormone production and act as a master regulator for energy and nutrient balance (Rosen & Spiegelman, 2014).

All fat cells mentioned above have roles to play throughout the body, but the cells that we are most interested in here are the **white ones**. Evolutionary-wise these are vital to our survival, as mentioned above, and they provide a limitless capacity for fat storage, particularly during times when food is plentiful. However, when food is scarce, metabolism changes and fatty acids are released from the cells and used by the brain and muscle (Ahima, 2006) thus ensuring we are still able to function.

The problem arises when healthy white fat cells become supercharged and this is sometimes known as "sick fat" or "angry fat" (Ahima, 2006; Bays, 2009). These cells then release a whole host of proteins, receptors, enzymes and transporters; they control the activity of sex hormones, inflammatory markers and immune responding cells; they increase inflammation and affect all the organs in the body via clever methods of cross talking (Ahima, 2006; Bays, 2009).

So what makes your fat angry?

Before we go any further we want to add a comment.

Fat cells are scientifically known as adipose cells (adipocytes) and a collection of these is known as adipose tissue. This tissue becomes an extremely complex organ that affects the whole body. We have simplified this explanation, which means a number of interacting factors have been omitted, as this is not the focus of our book. However, if you are interested in learning more about adipocyte biology please follow the references, which include some excellent reviews and articles.

What makes your fat angry?

1. **Happy fat cell.** Taking in food, toxins, etc. and storing them safely for a rainy day.

2. Excess food, toxins etc. go into mature fat cell.

3. Mature fat cell either needs to get bigger or sends a message to the body to send a new fat cell.

4. As food or toxins increase this recruitment of new fat cells either works well, okay or badly. This is where it starts to get *imbalanced.* If this system is slow or not working well, then new fat cells are not recruited and the fat cells we have already, just get bigger. Think of a balloon being blown up as much as possible. A 2010 study showed that overfeeding for just 8-weeks increased cell *number* above the waist but cell *size* below the waist (Tchoukalova et al., 2010).

5. These larger fat cells (which are now tissue) have reduced insulin sensitivity (frequently leading to sugar cravings), this happens in lean people too. These cells are an independent risk factor for type 2 diabetes and

people with these fat cells have poorer metabolic profiles than people with lots of smaller fat cells. This white fat tissue also becomes inflamed and filled with macrophages (a type of white blood cell that engulfs and digests cellular debris and foreign substances). In fact normal visceral fat (fat around the middle) has around 15% macrophages and in obesity it rises to as much as 60% (Odegaard & Chawla, 2012). And finally, although still up to now this is really only part of the story; fat cells are held together in a mesh-like bag (imagine satsuma's in a stringy bag). Current thinking is that flexible bags allow the fat cells to move freely around, while tough bags (imagine your satsuma's now in chicken wire) restrict the fat cells, meaning they can't store excess nutrients and this sets off stress-related pathways and inflammation. **Now we have angry fat.**

When the body has an excess number of these angry fat cells it no longer communicates the way that it should. These cells also affect the brain, the way the brain signals, and the way you respond to food or internal and external triggers (Meier & Gressner, 2004; Morton et al., 2014).

This brings us to location. Like buying a house or going on holiday, location matters. This is where the apple-shaped and pear-shaped scenario comes into play. The fat around our waist (apple) compared to the fat around our hips and thighs (pear) is far more metabolically active, it drains directly to the liver, meaning the liver has high concentrations of free fatty acids, metabolic and pro-inflammatory products. There is also a difference in oestrogen receptors, which may explain the abdominal weight-gain in menopausal women. When it is on your buttocks and thighs it is safe fat storage, when it's stored on your abdominal region, it isn't.

A 2010 study showed that overfeeding for just 8-weeks increased cell **number** above the waist but cell **size** below the waist (Tchoukalova et al., 2010).

What makes fat decide to go on your belly or your buttocks?

- Food choices
- Sleep
- Stress
- Genes – remember food also provides information to our genes
- Endocrine disruptors and toxins
- Intrauterine and childhood conditions
- Gut bacteria likely plays a role
  (Dhurander & Keith, 2014; Pestana et al., 2014)

Certain foods have been shown to change the function of the fat cells, support the fat cells to recruit new cells rather than stressing the large ones we already have, and therefore adapt the fat tissue (Baboota et al., 2013; Gonzalez-Castejon & Rodriguez-Casado, 2011; Rayalam et al., 2008; Williams et al., 2013; Bonet et al., 2015). Not only this, but because we are not just walking fat tissue, these foods have an important role to play within the rest of the body too. We have included these foods in our recipes and added them to our top twenty favourite foods in chapter 5.

By understanding this mechanism you understand where food comes into play. This is why nutrition professionals are focusing on food choices and food quality – we want to reduce the stress on the fat cell, reduce the inflammation and calm the system down, nourishing the cells in the body, and hence the person.

Generally patients mainly focus on losing weight, not always wanting to take on board, or maybe not fully understanding why or how certain foods help with weight-loss and other foods don't. The right foods help you lose weight.

Bariatric surgery is also known as a metabolic surgery as it affects many of the factors we've discussed above, including reducing inflammation. In fact 20% weight-loss from RYGB (Roux-en-Y gastric bypass) or LAGB (laparoscopic adjustable gastric band) positively affects inflammation, oral glucose tolerance and insulin sensitivity equally. This suggests that it's the weight-loss and changes in meal response that cause these changes, not the type of surgery (Bradley et al., 2012). However, if you still have excess weight, in particular abdominal weight, this scenario may have subsided but hasn't gone away.

Excess weight affects quality of life, from mental health, exercise ability, sleep quality, sexual function and more.

The good news is that change is possible. Nutrition and physical activity, independently or with medication or surgery, have been found to reduce white fat cells, along with reducing inflammatory markers and the risk factors associated with other lifestyle disease (Bays, 2009). The use of patient-centred strategies that encourage patients' active participation is likely to improve the post-operative care for band wearers (Moroshko et al., 2014).

What is your best weight?

Your best weight is what you wish to achieve while living the healthiest lifestyle you can truly enjoy.

Freedhoff & Sharma, 2010

2.5 Health implications of wearing a gastric band

There are additional health implications of wearing a band that we want to touch on, these include:

2.5.1 Reduced Vitamin & Mineral Status

Banding *reportedly* minimally affects vitamin and mineral absorption, however the research shows a real risk for nutritional deficiencies for the band wearer (Fish et al., 2010). These include deficiencies in Iron, Vitamin D, vitamin B1 and B12. Malnutrition has wider implications on overall health and should not be dismissed as a minor issue. This is covered in more depth in Nutrients – Chapter 6.

Malnutrition has wider implications on overall health and should not be dismissed as a minor issue.

2.5.2 Homocysteine

Homocysteine is a naturally occurring sulfur-containing amino acid, formed during the metabolism of methionine (an essential amino acid we get from dietary protein). We need folate, vitamin B12 and vitamin B6 to convert homocysteine back to methionine. If levels of these nutrients are low, the level of homocysteine increases. High homocysteine has been associated with many diseases including:

- Peripheral artery disease in men (Bertoia et al., 2014)

- Risk factor for reduced bone mineral density and increased risk of bone fracture and osteoporosis (Bailey et al., 2014; Enneman et al., 2014)
- Increased risk of dementia (Whalley et al., 2014)
- Higher prevalence of colour blindness in patients with diabetes (Sadiqulla et al., 2014)
- Obstructive sleep apnea (Niu et al., 2014)
- Kidney disease (Chao et al., 2014)

> **Gastric band patients have been found to have high homocysteine levels even when serum folate and B12 are not low (Dixon et al., 2001).**

According to Dixon et al. (2001), higher serum levels of folate and B12 are required to maintain homocysteine levels during weight-loss, even in those taking multivitamins, and the need for supplementation continues even when rate of weight-loss falls. Dixon states folate supplementation is essential at 400mcg daily in addition to dietary folate. As there is no malabsorption of B12 with a gastric band the recommended daily intake is sufficient. Gasteyger et al. (2006) found a 44.1% decline in folic acid levels in banded patients within two years of surgery. Changes in eating habits after surgery can result in low folate intake. This is particularly relevant for women who are planning future pregnancies, as folate is crucial in the prevention of neural tube defects in infants (Dixon et al., 2001).

Please read Chapter 7 – Supplements on the types of folate (folic acid) to be supplementing.

2.5.3 Calcium/Osteoporosis Risk

There is growing evidence that bariatric surgery, including gastric banding, has negative effects on bone density (Brozozowska et al., 2014) and increases risk of fracture (Nakamura et al., 2014).

2.5.4 Obesity and Bone Health

Obesity used to be considered good for the bones, due to the additional weight-bearing effects on the body. However, recent studies show that fat and bone metabolism are closely related, sharing regulatory locations (in the brain and the bone marrow). The relationship is complicated yet is affected by gender, affecting women more than men; hormonal status, affecting postmenopausal women more than pre-menopausal; and exercise, affecting those who are more sedentary than those who are more active (Cao, 2011; Reid, 2008; Soleymani, 2011).

Some bone loss may be inevitable as weight is lost, according to Von Mach et al. (2004), patients losing large amounts of body weight should be monitored regarding osteoporosis prevention.

We recommend having your bone turnover measured at frequent intervals by your bariatric team, or your Registered Nutritional Therapist. The frequency will depend on your results.

See chapter 6 for more information about the interactions between calcium, magnesium, vitamin D and Vitamin K2.

> The AACE/TOS/ASMBS 2013 Guidelines recommend bone density DXA scan at 2 years post-surgery for gastric band wearers.

2.5.5 Hyperparathyroidism

The parathyroid glands regulate the amount of calcium and phosphorus in the body so are important regarding osteoporosis risk. Elevated body mass index (BMI) and increasing degrees of obesity may be risk factors for vitamin D deficiency and secondary hyperparathyroidism (Fish et al., 2010). Vitamin D deficiency causes a long-standing low level of calcium in the blood, which stimulates the parathyroid glands to constantly try to raise your blood calcium level. This results in your parathyroid glands becoming enlarged. A study carried out in 2009 showed that 23.5% of their patients matched the criteria for hyperparathyroidism prior to surgery (Gimmel et al., 2009).

With secondary hyperparathyroidism, your calcium level is low so you may not develop all the symptoms mentioned below but you can develop problems with your bones. The increased level of parathyroid hormone in your blood causes large amounts of calcium to be released from your bones, causing your bones to become thin and weak (known as osteopenia) and making them more susceptible to breaks and fractures. If you experience any of the symptoms described below, we recommend you see your medical practitioner for blood tests on your calcium and parathyroid hormone levels.

Symptoms of hyperparathyroidism include:

- Tiredness
- Weak muscles
- Nausea and vomiting
- Lack of appetite
- Constipation
- Abdominal pain
- Thirst
- Frequent urination
- Depression

2.5.6 Dehydration/constipation

The small capacity of the stomach can make it difficult for band wearers to consume enough water, and patients may be at risk of dehydration (Harris & Barger, 2010). Fruit and vegetables, particularly those rich in fibre, are difficult for the banded patient to eat, which together with low fluid intake, may lead to constipation. Carrying a bottle of water and continuously sipping may help to prevent this. In chapter 5 we have included a list of fruits and vegetables that have high water content, which may be helpful.

Summary:

- ✓ What does health mean to you?
- ✓ Which area needs most attention – physical, mental or social?
- ✓ Health and disease are journeys, what is yours?
- ✓ Choose foods that calm down your fat cells and tissue.

✓ What is the best weight for you, living a healthy life that you truly enjoy?

✓ Consider the additional health implications of having a band.

✓ Check your levels of Vitamins D, B1, B12 and folate.

✓ Check your calcium and parathyroid hormone levels.

✓ Monitor for osteoporosis prevention – have your bone turnover measured.

Chapter 3

Considerations

> *You yourself, as much as anybody in the entire universe, deserve your love and affection.*
>
> Buddha

3.1 "I keep being told I'm fat, eat less, do more, that's all there is to it."

There is far more to excess weight than calories in, energy out. This chapter explains other factors that may have contributed to your weight gain and what you can do about it.

You may have had a band fitted some time ago and originally found you lost weight quite easily but have now plateaued. This chapter could explain why, as we cover common issues faced by our clients, including food and drink, thyroid function, allergies/intolerances, stress, hormones, blood sugar control, serotonin and depression, gut health and gut flora, movement and exercise, cognitive behaviour therapy, neuro-linguistic programming and hypnotherapy.

> **We are here to encourage eating, but eating to fuel your body, your mind and giving you the nutrients you need to be healthy.**

Being overweight and then obese does not just happen overnight and we've already briefly discussed some of the reasons why this is happening. Food and exercise are of course important, but hormones and inflammatory changes that occur in the body when it is obese change the way your hormone messengers communicate with one another, your digestive system, liver, immune system, and brain (Meier & Gressner, 2004). Your body is not talking in the same way as a muscly lean body, which is really important for you to know.

There are some things which are associated with being obese which do not go away after having a gastric band fitted – so if you are thinking about having a band, or have a band and still are not feeling 'quite right' – or even thinking about having your band removed, then you may first like to consider these:

3.2 Overview diagram of other considerations:

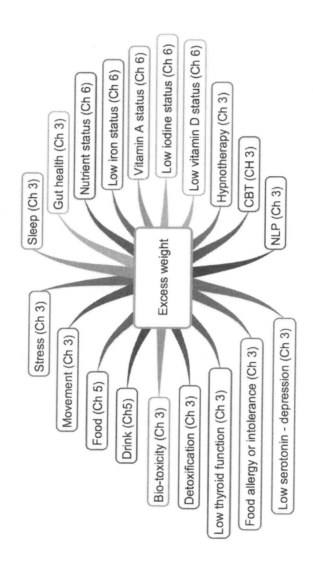

3.3 Food and Drink

Eating and drinking should be an enjoyable experience; however what you eat or drink has a huge impact on your health, mood and weight. Chapter 5 is dedicated to eating and we share with you the best options for food and drink.

3.4 Low Thyroid Function

Hypothyroidism is the term given for an under-active thyroid gland. The thyroid is a butterfly-shaped endocrine gland located in the front of the neck whose job is to regulate the body's use of energy and keep all our organs working properly.

Hypothyroidism means the thyroid gland isn't producing enough of the hormone thyroxine (T4), so there's too little in the blood to keep the body running as it should.

Thyroid hormones are essential and primary regulators of the body's metabolism. Imbalances can affect virtually every metabolic process in the body, exerting significant effects on mood and energy levels.

Thyroid hormones are carried in the blood to every tissue in the body so when levels are too low the whole body's processes slow down, which is why there are so many varied symptoms. If you suffer with some of the symptoms below, do the Barnes Temperature Test below or consider having a thyroid test.

3.4.1 Common symptoms of low thyroid function

- Mental fatigue
- Depression
- Irritability
- Slow heart rate
- High cholesterol
- Constipation
- Poor digestion and bloating
- Increased susceptibility to colds
- Feeling run down
- Weight gain and hard to lose weight
- Feeling cold
- Premenstrual syndrome
- Infertility
- Less interest in sex
- Thick tongue
- Goiter
- Course, thinning or brittle hair
- Pale, dry or flaky skin

3.4.2 Thyroid Home Test

You will need:

1 digital basal thermometer (available online for around £4)

1 pen and this chart

Method:

1. Before going to bed place thermometer within easy reach of the bed along the pen and the chart.

2. When you wake up in the morning, **before getting up**, put the thermometer under your armpit and lie quietly until it beeps.

3. Note the temperature and write it down on the chart.

4. Repeat this process until the chart is complete.

Menstruating women should make a note on the chart of the days of their cycle as body temperatures fluctuate during the cycle.

Day 1	Day 2	Day 3	Day 4	Day 5	Day 6	Day 7	Day 8	Day 9	Day 10
Day 11	Day 12	Day 13	Day 14	Day 15	Day 16	Day 17	Day 18	Day 19	Day 20
Day 21	Day 22	Day 23	Day 24	Day 25	Day 26	Day 27	Day 28	Day 29	Day 30

If the average reading is 36.5°C or lower your thyroid gland is under functioning and you are possibly hypothyroid. If the average reading is 36.9°C or higher you may have hyperthyroidism (overactive thyroid) or an infection.

Your average temperature should fall between 36.6-36.8°C. If it is outside this range, it may be advisable to get your thyroid checked via your GP or a Total Thyroid Assessment by a Registered Nutritional Therapist.

In many cases, a low temperature will not necessarily indicate a condition which would be medically diagnosed as an underactive thyroid, but may still benefit from nutritional support.

3.5 Food Allergy and Intolerance

Over 60 years ago (1947) Randolph presented his research on "Masked Food Allergy as a factor in the development and persistence of obesity", yet the link between obesity and food allergies is still controversial.

Over the past couple of decades there have been increases in both obesity and allergies, particularly in children – and this may be why the majority of studies involve children rather than adults. So what is the connection and does it have anything to do with you?

When the body gets over a certain weight the fat cells start to change. They may change in size or number as discussed in chapter 2. What is important is that the messages they send out change. They signal to the rest of the immune system that the body is inflamed; this makes the immune system work harder to try and reduce the inflammation.

When someone eats a food that they react to, a similar system is deployed in the body, messages are sent to try and reduce the inflammatory response to a food that the body has recognised as a foreign object.

So certain parts of the underlying mechanism appear to be similar between weight gain and inflammation, and systemic inflammation is likely to be a factor. Scientifically it would be good to know which tends to come first, the food allergy or intolerance, or the weight gain, although it is most likely that this will depend on the individual.

3.5.1 Signs of food allergy or intolerance

- Food addiction
- Mouth ulcers
- Burning mouth
- Nausea and indigestion
- Heartburn
- Stomach ulcers
- Duodenal ulcers
- Diarrhoea
- Constipation
- Irritable Bowel Syndrome
- Crohn's Disease
- Bloating and wind
- Itchiness
- Muscular aches
- Aching joints
- Rheumatoid arthritis and other forms of arthritis
- Backache
- Irregular heartbeat
- Chest pain
- Headaches
- Migraines
- Mental symptoms – this may include drowsiness, dizziness or lack of concentration.

- Red itchy or watery eyes
- Bedwetting or incontinence
- Water retention
- Epileptic fits
- Flushing, sweating or chilling
- Fatigue
- Hypoglycaemia (low blood sugar)
- Premenstrual tension

It may be advisable to have an allergy, immunology test (there are different types of food allergy and intolerance tests available) or follow an elimination diet. It is recommended that this is carried out alongside a qualified health practitioner.

3.6 Stress

When faced with a stressful situation, your body releases the chemicals cortisol, adrenaline and noradrenaline to invoke the 'fight or flight' response. The problem is that if you can't fight or escape the situation, such as being stressed at work or when driving, these chemicals are not used and stay in the body. A build-up of adrenaline and noradrenaline increases blood pressure, heart rate, the amount you sweat, and reduces digestion. Cortisol prompts the release of glucose into the bloodstream, and if this glucose is not used to produce energy, the body will store it as fat, usually around your midriff.

Sugar, refined foods and stimulants such as caffeine, alcohol and nicotine, can lead to or increase feelings of stress.

It has been proposed that obesity may be considered a maladaptation to stress exposure, with stress leading to hyper-activation of the hypothalamic-pituitary-adrenal (HPA) axis, resulting in higher-than-normal cortisol levels (Vicenatti et al., 2014).

Blood sugar imbalance and weight gain

Stress can lead to cravings for sweet foods and stimulants, setting up a vicious cycle of blood sugar surges and dips with the corresponding surges in insulin release when blood sugar is high and cortisol release when blood sugar is low. These energy highs and lows lead to tiredness, more energy slumps, headaches, poor concentration and restless sleep which all leave you feeling more and more tired and in need of the sugar or caffeine to keep going.

Reduced absorption of nutrients and lowered nutrient status

When stressed, the body slows digestion as energy is diverted elsewhere, which may lead to digestive problems including indigestion, constipation, diarrhoea, symptoms of IBS and increased intestinal permeability which causes inflammation in the gut and possible subsequent food intolerances.

Poor digestion leads to poor absorption of nutrients, so while more and more fat is deposited around your middle, you're actually becoming malnourished, resulting in less energy and more fatigue, a weakened immune system and altered metabolism.

While compromising your digestion (and absorption), stress increases your needs for vitamins and minerals, in particular the B vitamins, vitamin C and other antioxidants, calcium and magnesium.

Hormone Imbalance

If you're chronically stressed, this sustained release of adrenaline and cortisol can lead to hormone imbalances as well as adrenal exhaustion, which can affect your thyroid, causing a slow in your metabolism and induce weight gain, reduce sex drive, affect fertility and result in extreme tiredness. Neurotransmitters in the brain can also be affected, resulting in depression, poor concentration and memory, mood swings, anger, irritability and disturbed sleep.

Cardiovascular problems

As mentioned above, adrenaline increases your blood pressure and heart rate, so long periods of stress coupled with a high sugar/stimulant diet can lead to many problems such as cardiovascular disease, insulin resistance and diabetes.

Tension is who you think you should be.
Relaxation is who you are.

Chinese Proverb

If you suffer with some of the symptoms below, complete the Adrenal Health Questionnaire.

3.6.1 Common Symptoms of Stress

- Cravings
- Frequent illness
- Weight gain
- Low libido
- Fertility problems
- Depression
- Poor memory
- Mood swings
- Anger
- Irritability
- Low energy
- Food intolerances
- IBS
- Disturbed sleep
- Poor concentration
- High blood pressure
- Indigestion
- Constipation
- Diarrhoea
- Headaches
- Fatigue

It's not stress that kills us, it's our reaction to it.

Hans Seyle

3.6.2 Adrenal Health Questionnaire

Key:
0 – No or do not have the symptom
1 – Yes or symptom is mild/rarely occurs (once a month or less)
2 – Symptom is moderate or occasionally occurs (weekly)
3 – Symptom is severe or frequently occurs (daily)

Please complete swiftly, without too much deliberation

1. Tend to be a 'night person'......................................
2. Difficulty falling asleep...
3. Slow starter in the morning....................................
4. Keyed up, trouble calming down............................
5. High blood pressure (normal 120/80)....................
6. Headache after exercising..
7. Feeling wired or jittery if drinking coffee.............
8. Clench or grind teeth...
9. Calm on the outside, troubled inside......................
10. Chronic low back pain, worse with fatigue...........
11. Become dizzy when standing up suddenly............
12. Difficult maintaining osteopathic treatment.......
13. Pain after osteopathic treatment..........................
14. Arthritic tendencies...
15. Crave salty foods..
16. Salt foods before tasting..
17. Perspire easily...
18. Chronic fatigue, or get drowsy often...................
19. Afternoon yawning...
20. Afternoon headache..
21. Asthma, wheezing, difficulty breathing...............
22. Pain on inner side of the knee..............................
23. Tendency to 'shin splints'.......................................
24. Tendency to need to wear sunglasses...................
25. Allergies and/or hives..
26. Weakness, dizziness..
                                                Total...............................

> **If the total score is 25 or above, it may be advisable to get your adrenal health checked via your GP or an Adrenal Stress Profile arranged by a Registered Nutritional Therapist.**

3.7 Low Serotonin and Depression

Serotonin is a neurotransmitter that is involved in feelings of happiness or wellbeing, gut motility, memory, learning and regulation of sleep and appetite.

It acts on the brain but is primarily found and produced in the gut. People with low levels of serotonin have been found to have lower moods, whereas those with higher levels are found to be more positive. Serotonin levels and depression are closely linked and there is an undisputed reciprocal link between depression and obesity. Obesity has been found to increase the risk of depression, and depression has been found to be predictive of developing obesity (Luppino et al., 2010).

Increasing feelings of happiness are important as they improve overall well-being as well as health outcomes.

> *There is a morning inside you waiting to burst open into light.*
>
> Rumi

Raising Serotonin Naturally

1) Diet – increasing foods which contain tryptophan – i.e. good quality protein – at every meal.

2) Exercise – increases brain serotonin function and increases tryptophan – tryptophan is needed to make serotonin, so we have a double whammy! It is well known that exercise improves mood. So find something you like doing.

3) Exposure to bright light – this is a standard treatment for seasonal depression but studies have also found it to be beneficial in non-seasonal depression and depressed pregnant women.

4) Self induced changes in mood change serotonin synthesis – so thinking happy thoughts can change the levels and influence your moods. If you are struggling with finding this in yourself then try reading encouraging and positive books, or watching uplifting films, listening to positive and lively music – alternatively seek support from a professional to help give you a kick start (Young, 2007).

Diet, Obesity and Depression

Low quality diets are categorised as being LOW in fruit and vegetables, low in fibre and low in protein from nuts and plant sources – and HIGH in saturated fats, trans fats, alcohol and sodium. Diets like the above are associated with obesity and depression (Appelhans et al., 2012).

3.8 *Sleep*

Sleep, weight gain, and resetting circadian rhythm

> **Sleep, despite being a sedentary activity, may protect the most against weight gain.**

The evidence is clear that people who sleep less, either through short sleep duration or disturbed sleep, have an increased risk of obesity (Beccuti & Pannain, 2011). Short-term partial sleep restriction decreases glucose tolerance, elevates cortisol concentrations, decreases leptin (the satiety hormone), increases the appetite-stimulating hormone ghrelin, and increases hunger and appetite (Chatput et al., 2010). Being tired could also make it more difficult to get sufficient exercise.

Both adults and children have shorter bedtimes than a few decades ago and this trend of shorter sleep duration has developed over the same time period as the dramatic increase in obesity prevalence (Van Cauter & Knutson, 2008). The impact of short sleep duration and quality on the risk of obesity may be greater in children (Van Cauter & Knutson, 2008).

Sleep resets your circadian rhythm, the body's 'clock'. The circadian rhythm controls functions such as when you sleep and wake, your body temperature, the balance of body fluids, and appetite. Keeping regular meal and exercise times will help steady your body clock and sleep pattern. Ideally go to bed and get up at the same time each day (including weekends) and make sure the room you sleep in is dark and quiet (no televisions, computers or mobile phones).

It may be ironic, but sleep, despite being a sedentary activity, may protect the most against weight gain. Going to bed early enough to ensure a good 8 hours sleep may have a significant impact on not only how you feel but also on your ability to control your weight.

3.9 Bio-toxicity and Detoxification

It is beyond the scope of this book to discuss in depth the issues surrounding the impact that our increasingly toxic environment is having on our wellbeing, and in particular on serious epidemic health conditions including cancer, cardiovascular disease, respiratory health, infertility, diabetes, and obesity. This section has been provided to give the reader an overview and to highlight another factor that needs considering with regards to weight-loss and weight management.

Chemicals that affect our hormones, metabolism and weight control mechanisms are known as endocrine disrupting hormones and many of these act as obesogens.

Obesogens are chemical pollutants that are able to promote obesity by changing metabolism, disrupting appetite controls, promoting bigger fat cells (discussed in chapter 2) and promoting more fat cells during development, childhood and adulthood.

Grun, 2010

Our environment is not only under threat from being over-populated but also from an abundance of man-made toxic chemicals that we are all being constantly exposed to. There are more than 80,000 chemicals on the market today, found in furniture, toys, processed food, food packaging and personal products, and only a tiny percentage of these have been tested for health effects (Attar & Bowman, 2014).

Air pollution is also a risk factor for obesity and obese individuals are more vulnerable to the harmful effects of air pollution (Limaye & Salvi, 2014).

Toxins affect the hormones that regulate weight, they alter our appetite and how satisfied we feel after a meal. Toxins also trigger inflammation and damage mitochondria affecting our energy levels (Hyman, 2007).

A study was recently carried out on patients undergoing bariatric surgery and the team found that persistent organic pollutants (POP's) were mainly stored in abdominal fat (remember the apple shape we discussed in chapter 2). With people having higher levels the older they were, and higher levels as well in those who had been obese for longer. Not only that, the POP level correlated with hypertension, dysglycemia (discussed in chapter 5) and cardiovascular risk. Of more interest for patients when it comes to weight-loss, they found that the higher the POP level the less weight-loss occurred, especially in older patients (Pestana et al., 2014).

The higher the POP levels, the lower the weight-loss.

We recommend this *four-step* process:
1. Test for toxins and detoxification function
2. Remove and reduce toxin intake
3. Improve elimination
4. Use diet and lifestyle to reduce toxic load and support detoxification pathways

1. Test for toxins

Liver function can be measured by your GP or health professional. For a further personalised approach it is worth considering having a more comprehensive assessment of toxic elements such as heavy metals, organophosphates, moulds or hidden infections measured either through your GP, if they are familiar with these testing options, or with a Registered Nutritional Therapist.

For an indication of how well your body's detoxification process is working, complete the Biotoxicity Symptom Questionnaire below.

2. Remove and reduce toxin intake

Avoid exposure to heavy metals, electromagnetic radiation, allergens and petrochemicals. A Western diet that is energy dense, high in processed foods and saturated fat increases our exposure to obesogens. Sharpe & Drake (2013) reported that diet is a predominate source of obesogens, their comments are based on studies showing that around 95% of our exposure to Bisphenol A comes from food (Kang et al., 2006) and that by swapping packaged foods for the same ingredients that were freshly sourced and unpackaged, Bisphenol A urinary levels were reduced by up to 66% and diethylhexyl phthalate (one of the most common phthalates) was reduced by more than 50% (Rudel et al., 2011).

3. Improve elimination

Drink 6-8 glasses of filtered water a day.

Ensure you have regular bowel movements, ideally one per day.

Sweat through exercise or by using a steam room or sauna.

4. Use diet and lifestyle to reduce toxic load and support detoxification pathways.

It is recommended that you focus on freshly sourced organic produce, emphasising fruits, vegetables, whole grains, beans and pulses. Cruciferous vegetables including cabbage, broccoli, collards, kale, Brussel sprouts, Chinese cabbage, rocket, watercress, mustard greens and turnips, along with turmeric and curry, green tea, eggs, garlic, and onions are the most effective foods to support detoxification (Hyman, 2010). A large number of the recipes provided in this book have been chosen to support liver function and optimise natural detoxification pathways.

3.9.1 Biotoxicity Symptom Questionnaire

Rate each of the following symptoms based upon your typical health profile:

Point Scale

0 – Never or almost never have the symptoms
1 – Occasionally has it, effect is not severe
2 – Occasionally has it, effect is severe
3 – Frequently has it, effect is not severe
4 – Frequently has it, effect is severe

Add up the numbers to arrive at a total for each section, and then add the totals for each section to arrive at the grand total. If any individual section total is 10 or more, or the grand total is **50** or more, you may benefit from a detoxification programme.

DIGESTIVE
— NAUSEA OR VOMITING
— DIARRHEA
— CONSTIPATION
— BLOATED FEELING
— BELCHING, PASSING GAS
— HEARTBURN
— TOTAL

EMOTIONS
— MOOD SWINGS
— ANXIETY, FEAR, NERVOUS
— ANGER, IRRITABILITY
— DEPRESSION
— TOTAL

EYES
— WATERY, ITCHY EYES
— SWOLLEN, REDDENED OR STICKY EYELIDS
— DARK CIRCLES UNDER EYES
— BLURRED / TUNNEL VISION
— TOTAL

LUNGS
— CHEST CONGESTION
— ASTHMA, BRONCHITIS
— SHORTNESS OF BREATH
— DIFFICULTY BREATHING
— TOTAL

EARS
— ITCHY EARS
— EARACHES, EAR INFECTION
— DRAINAGE FROM EAR
— RINGING IN EARS, HEARING LOSS
— TOTAL

ENERGY/ACTIVITY
— FATIGUE, SLUGGISHNESS
— APATHY, SLUGGISHNESS
— HYPERACTIVITY
— RESTLESSNESS
— TOTAL

HEAD
— HEADACHES
— FAINTNESS
— DIZZINESS
— INSOMNIA
— TOTAL

MIND
— POOR MEMORY
— CONFUSION
— POOR CONCENTRATION
— POOR COORDINATION
— DIFFICULTY MAKING DECISIONS
— STUTTERING, STAMMERING
— SLURRED SPEECH
— LEARNING DISABILITIES
— TOTAL

MOUTH/THROAT
— CHRONIC COUGHING
— GAGGING, NEED TO CLEAR THROAT
— SORE THROAT, HOARSE
— SWOLLEN OR DISCOLORED TONGUE, GUMS, LIPS
— CANKER SORES
— TOTAL

SKIN
— ACNE
— HIVES, RASHES, DRY SKIN
— HAIR LOSS
— FLUSHING OR HOT FLASHES
— EXCESSIVE SWEATING
— TOTAL

JOINT/MUSCLES
— PAIN OR ACHES IN JOINTS
— ARTHRITIS
— STIFF, LIMITED MOVEMENT
— PAIN, ACHES IN MUSCLES
— WEAKNESS OR TIREDNESS
— TOTAL

NOSE
— STUFFY NOSE
— SINUS PROBLEMS
— HAY FEVER
— SNEEZING ATTACKS
— EXCESSIVE MUCUS
— TOTAL

HEART
— SKIPPED HEARTBEATS
— RAPID HEARTBEATS
— CHEST PAIN
— TOTAL

WEIGHT
— BINGE EATING / DRINKING
— CRAVING CERTAIN FOODS
— EXCESSIVE WEIGHT GAIN
— COMPULSIVE EATING
— WATER RETENTION
— UNDERWEIGHT
— TOTAL

OTHER
— FREQUENT ILLNESS
— FREQUENT / URGENT URINATION
— GENITAL ITCH DISCHARGE
— TOTAL

_____ **GRAND TOTAL**

Source: Center For Alternative Medicine

3.10 *Gut Health*

We have previously mentioned how an overweight body is not speaking the same language as a lean body. This is not only due to adaptations in fat cells and hormone signalling (discussed in Chapter 2) but also due to differences in gut micro-biome (the bacteria in the gastrointestinal tract).

There are many factors that affect our micro-biome; these include genes, physiology, early life experiences, age, and diet (Conterno et al., 2011; Di Baise et al., 2012). Changes also occur during pregnancy, with antibiotic use, jet lag, shift-work, laughter (Kimata, 2010), exercise, and after weight-loss surgery (Deizenne et al., 2011; Di Baise et al., 2012; Thaiss et al., 2014). Which is one reason your band might feel different when you are stressed or at altitude such as when flying or skiing.

The gut micro-biome and its ability to regulate body weight have been under increasing scrutiny. Studies have confirmed that alterations in the composition of our gut flora are associated with obesity (Devaraj et al., 2013; Ley, 2010). It appears the gut micro-biome of obese individuals is more efficient at extracting calories from food than lean people, and these bacteria stimulate glucose and fat production (Mutzel, 2014).

Everything we eat has an effect on our micro-biome and a high-fat low-fibre Western-style diet dramatically impacts the gut microbiota (Conterno et al., 2011). A diet high in fat and refined carbohydrates promotes inflammation and feeds 'bad' bacteria, which reduces the body's ability to burn fat as fuel. Whereas by choosing anti-inflammatory high fibre foods such as fruit and vegetables we feed the 'good' bacteria and can help the body switch to burning fat as its primary fuel.

> *Changing diet manipulates the micro-biome, alters gut function and metabolism and therefore promotes healthy weight-loss.*
>
> Mullin & Delzenne, 2014

Pre and Pro-biotics

Pre-biotics are foods that feed our 'friendly bacteria', improve glucose tolerance, and reduce inflammation. These include asparagus, bananas, chicory, Jerusalem artichokes, leeks, garlic, and onion.

Probiotics adapt the gut micro-biome and include a variety of species but the most commonly known are Lactobacillus and Bifidobacteria. Probiotics are found in dietary supplements or in fermented foods such as unpasteurised sauerkraut, apple cider vinegar, 'live' yogurt, kefir and miso soup.

A number of studies show probiotic intervention has beneficial effects on obesity, by reducing the size of the fat cell, helping improve insulin sensitivity and accelerating weight-loss (Ley, 2010; Wolf & Lorenz, 2012; DiBaise et al., 2012).

Current research is focusing on the effects of antibiotics and obesity. There are a number of studies showing an increased risk in childhood obesity and antibiotic use. If you have been a long-term user of antibiotics it may be worth having a full digestive screen carried out to assess your gut micro-biome.

3.11 Movement

We are not suggesting that you need to go mad and put your name down for a marathon, even though you could, but before that, just move "your booty" – starting off with walking, dancing, gardening, more 'up-and-down-the-stairs', and keep a record of what you do, slowly increasing it. Exercise makes you feel alive and, whether it is part of your pre or post-op plan, it is vital to your overall wellbeing.

The handbook, "Exercise is Medicine" summarises a number of studies and recommendations for using exercise for weight-loss, weight maintenance and to prevent weight gain. The authors report that training has positive effects on the development and symptoms of obesity, physical fitness and strength, and enhances quality of life. Without even changing any dietary aspects 13 – 26 hours of physical activity (measured as MET-hours) a week leads to a decrease in total and abdominal fat and improves metabolic function. Current evidence shows that abdominal fat loss with increased activity is proportional to overall fat loss (Blair et al., 2011).

> **13 MET hours is equivalent to walking at a 4-mile an hour pace (6.4km/hr) for 150 minutes a week. To keep this simple we commonly recommend brisk walking 3 times a week for an hour each time. Of course you need to work out what fits in with your new lifestyle.**

We recommend working with a professional who routinely uses exercise prescriptions as a form of treatment. Training plans should be personalised and will differ depending on your fitness level, BMI and other comorbidities.

Not just your body, what about your mind as well?

The mind and body are one, if you are thinking about moving your body why not also consider working with your mind? Hypnotherapy, Neuro Linguistic Programming and Cognitive Behaviour Therapy all focus on the mind and behaviour.

In teenagers and adults, emotional eating is associated with an increased consumption of fatty foods and a higher BMI (Cartwright et al., 2003; Konttinen et al., 2010) and as discussed above those who are sleep deprived and tired are more likely to be overweight or obese (Patel & Hu, 2008; Chaput et al., 2011).

People don't always need advice. Sometimes all they really need is a hand to hold, an ear to listen, and a heart to understand them.

Unknown

3.12 Cognitive Behaviour Therapy (CBT)

CBT is a form of counselling that helps to change how you think ('cognitive') and what you do ('behaviour'). The basis of CBT is to change the way a person thinks about failure, defeat, loss and helplessness and has been shown to help with many different types of problems including eating disorders, stress and depression.

Your GP may refer you to a therapist if they believe it will be helpful or you can find a registered therapist by looking on: www.babcp.com

3.13 Neuro Linguistic Programming (NLP)

NLP centres on communication and change.

Neuro – NLP is based on the idea that you experience the world through your senses and translate this into thoughts, both conscious and subconscious. This effects your emotions, behaviour and physiology.

Linguistic – is the way you use language to express these experiences to others. NLP is about the words you speak and the body language you use and how these may influence your experiences.

Programming – consists of your internal processing and strategies, how you make decisions or solve problems, learn, evaluate or get results. NLP shows you how to recode experiences and organise thoughts so that you can get the outcomes you want (Ready & Burton, 2011).

To find an NLP practitioner or to learn more visit: www.anlp.org

3.14 Hypnotherapy

Hypnotherapy addresses the unconscious brain in order to re-programme the conscious brain and can de-condition established habits, thereby facilitating an unconscious re-learning process (British Society of Clinical Hypnosis).

Hypnotherapy is medically accepted and could benefit the following: unwanted habits, weight control/healthy eating, boost self-confidence, achieving potential, emotional problems, compulsions, sleep problems, inhibitions, reduce stress plus many others (listed by the British Society of Clinical Hypnosis).

Hypnotherapy may benefit those who find it difficult to give up certain foods, lifestyles, behaviours and addictions.

To find a registered hypnotherapist visit: www.bsch.org.uk.

Summary:

✓ There are many factors to consider when it comes to weight-loss and weight maintenance. What factors most affect you?

✓ What is the quality of your food and drink? What can you upgrade or change?

✓ Is your thyroid working properly – have you used the temperature test?

✓ Could food allergy/intolerance be a factor – check the signs and symptoms to see if you would benefit from testing or need to seek further advice.

✓ How are your stress levels? Complete the adrenal health questionnaire to initially assess your adrenals.

✓ Are you getting enough sleep?

✓ Does your body detoxify efficiently? Complete the biotoxicity questionnaire and seek further support if indicated.

✓ How is your digestion? Could you have imbalanced gut flora?

✓ What exercise and movement are you doing or willing to try?

✓ Could CBT, NLP or hypnotherapy be helpful?

✓ Consider working with other health professionals including movement, behaviour, re-programming and hypnotherapy specialists.

For Food and Drink please see chapter 5.

For these other considerations please see Chapter 6:

- Vitamin A status
- Vitamin D status
- Iodine status
- Iron status
- Nutrient status

Chapter 4

Fertility, Preconception and Pregnancy

> *Pregnancy is a process that invites you to surrender to the unseen force behind all life.*
>
> Judy Ford

4.1 Obesity and Fertility

There are a wide variety of factors involved in preconception, fertility status, becoming pregnant and maintaining a pregnancy. These variants include our inherited genetics, past and present gene-environment-nutrient interactions, our unique anatomy and physiology, age, hormone profiles, immune systems, toxicity levels, stress levels, gut flora, support networks and far more. It is outside the remit of this chapter to discuss all of the above, hence an overview, specifically relevant to gastric band wearers, has been provided.

We strongly recommend that you work with a multi-disciplinary team throughout your pregnancy. If seeking advice from elsewhere ensure your primary health care provider is fully aware of everyone else you are working with, and ensure you share information.

4.1.1 In Women

Obesity has negative effects on fertility as it affects the menstrual cycle, the quality of oocytes (eggs) and the receptivity of the uterine lining (Jungheim et al., 2013). It also reduces ovulation frequency, which may be due to high insulin levels or poor liver function, both of which can lead to imbalances of sex hormones, as well as other complex factors (Kominiarek, 2011).

A survey conducted in 2010 with 1,538 females found 42% of women who tried to become pregnant before bariatric surgery had experienced infertility (Gosman et al., 2010).

Hormone profiles have been shown in some cases to change after weight-loss surgery but the evidence is still inconclusive as to whether this applies to everyone or just certain individuals.

Data indicates improved fertility in women after surgery (Gracia et al., 2014), however current recommendations suggest that women should not be advised to have weight-loss surgery solely to increase their chances of pregnancy (Sheiner et al., 2013).

4.1.2 In Men

Obesity has nearly tripled in reproductive aged men in the last 30 years; this coincides with an increase in male infertility (Palmer et al., 2012).

Obesity in men alters sex hormone profiles, and affects sperm count, concentration and quality. There is a higher chance of having DNA fragmentation; this may lead to reduced fertility and a higher incidence of partners having a miscarriage (Du Plessis et al., 2010). Poor sperm quality also affects the health cues that are passed onto the next generation. Animal models show these affected sperm may pass on an increased chance of autism, diabetes, and obesity in offspring (Palmer et al., 2012).

> *Men who lose weight through diet and exercise can improve their sex hormone profile, erectile function, sexual response and sperm parameters.*
>
> Du Plessis et al., 2010, Kasturi et al., 2008; Isidori et al., 1999; Chavarro et al., 2009; Hanna et al., 2009

Weight-loss surgery shows promising results in restoring sex hormone levels, yet there is very limited data with regards to the quality of sperm afterwards. In 2005, six men who were fertile before surgery were left azospermic (no sperm) after Roux-en-Y (roo-en-why) gastric bypass (RYGB) (di Frega et al., 2005). A 2012 paper (Sermondale et al., 2012) discusses three male patients where sperm quality was severely worsened after bariatric surgery. In one case the sperm quality improved again after 2 years. Lazeros et al., (2012) reported on two cases where, again, sperm parameters worsened. Reis et al., (2012) showed in their group of 20 men who had gastric bypass that their sperm was not affected. Legro et al., (2014) studied six men (again RYGB) and they found sperm parameters were reduced but not significantly. The studies mentioned above suggest that dramatic weight-loss may be detrimental to sperm production and therefore fertility.

Bariatric surgery should not be recommended as a solution to obesity-linked infertility (Du Plessis et al., 2010) and physicians should be informing their patients of the impacts of surgery on their fertility status (Reis & Dias, 2012).

We were unable to find specific studies on gastric banding and semen parameters. We therefore highly recommend you have your semen assessed prior to conceiving.

What about sexual satisfaction?

Women

A 2011 study found that sexual dysfunction decreased in women after having a gastric band fitted (Bond et al., 2011). This is supported by a 2014 study showing improvements in sexual function and sexual psychological status in a group of 106 women (Sarwer et al., 2014).

Men

In men we were unable to find any studies focusing on gastric band wearers but other weight-loss surgeries have been investigated and show an overall improved sexual function (Hammoud et al., 2009). A small 2014 study with 30 men showed again an increase in all areas of sexual function except male orgasm (Efthymiou et al., 2014).

4.2 Obesity, pregnancy and gastric banding safety

The number of women of reproductive age who have a gastric band fitted has increased significantly in recent years, it's deemed a safe and well-tolerated procedure for both the mother and the newborn (Skull et al., 2004; Bar-Zohar et al., 2006; Vrebosch et al., 2012).

Complications such as hypertension and gestational diabetes are significantly reduced (Skull et al., 2004), as are pre-eclampsia, emergency caesarean section, preterm birth, spontaneous abortion and newborns that are large for gestational age (Bar-Zohar et al., 2006; Vrebosch et al., 2012). However these complications are still higher than when compared with normal weight women (Vrebosch et al., 2012).

One area of concern is the increased numbers of women after weight-loss surgery (including banding) giving birth to small for gestational age babies (Kjær et al., 2013). Babies that are small for their gestational age are at higher risk of metabolic syndrome, cardiovascular disease and diabetes in later life (Marchal & Jaquet, 2004). The scientists that carried out the above study recommend maternal nutritional deficiencies to be monitored during pregnancy (Kjær et al., 2013). It is worth noting that the risks were higher in the group of bypass patients compared to those with bands. Women with gastric bands have a lower weight gain during pregnancy (Lapolla et al., 2010). However, this does depend partly on how much the band is loosened or not (Pilone et al., 2014).

Although there are no significant differences in mother or baby complications all pregnancies following bariatric surgery should still be managed as a high-risk pregnancy by a multidisciplinary team.

It is essential that you are part of a supportive team, if you are not, find someone who you enjoy working with. Your team is there to support you and your pregnancy. Ultimately however we are responsible for our own health – finding healthcare providers that encourage and motivate us in a positive way, helps us help ourselves.

4.3 Pre-conception Testing Recommendations

Gastric band wearers are less affected nutritionally than those who have had RYGB procedure, however, it is recommended that prior to conception you have a nutritional screen carried out (American College of Obstetrics and Gynecologists, 2013). When optimal levels are achieved, then you should plan to conceive. Once conception has occurred testing should be continued each trimester (Chilelli et al., 2014).

> **Your aim is to be optimally nourished prior to conception.**

The tests we recommended include:

✓ A full blood count
✓ A complete nutrient screen including vitamins A, D and K, B1 and B12
✓ Calcium
✓ Iodine
✓ Homocysteine
✓ Gastrointestinal screen

These should be on top of the tests that are carried out as part of your routine checkups. Tests should include:

A full blood count, to include **iron levels** and **red blood cell folate**. This test is commonly used to assess a person's general health and is commonly taken during pregnancy.

Vitamin A is essential for the human body but more so during times of growth and development. Your baby needs vitamin A not only for growth but also for development of eyes, skin, organs including the heart, and mucus membranes. Vitamin A is essential for immune functions and evaluation is recommended (Chagas et al., 2013). Vitamin A is particularly important in the second and third trimester of pregnancy for normal foetal lung development, and the pregnant mother's status affects the stores of the foetus (Kaska et al., 2013)

Vitamin D regulates cell growth and differentiation and therefore may have a crucial role to play in the development of the foetus. It is needed in pregnancy for your baby's bone development.

The effect of maternal vitamin D deficiency (or adequacy) may differ according to the season. In the UK, for example, levels are lowest in January, February and March, and this may affect levels in the foetus (Foss, 2009).

Vitamin D deficiency has been implicated in gestational diabetes and pre-eclampsia (Martineau & Khan, 2014), preterm birth and bacterial vaginosis (Skowrońska-Jóźwiak et al., 2014) and may also be involved in recurrent pregnancy loss (Ota et al., 2014). Therefore, monitoring of vitamin D status is recommended (Medeiros et al., 2013).

Vitamin K deficiency can present a serious health risk to pregnant women and their babies that may lead to haemorrhage, especially in newborns. Requirements also increase during pregnancy and deficiencies are more likely to occur during this period (Shahrook et al., 2014). Excessive vomiting, common in pregnant band wearers, may lead to a higher risk of deficiency (Kominiarek, 2011; Kaska et al., 2013).

B vitamins should be measured, as they are commonly deficient in the bariatric patient. All B vitamins are essential for cell division, needed to make your baby. They also create new blood cells and help the brain and nervous system develop fully. Folate (B9) is passed on in breast milk and increases the risk in the infant of lowered immunity, slow speech, poor muscle and weight, poor sleep, gastrointestinal problems, mood dysfunction and fatigue (Lynch, 2014). See Chapter 6 for more details about folate and folic acid.

Calcium is required for the development of your baby's bone, heart and nervous system. Inadequate intake may result in maternal bone loss, poor mineralisation of foetal skeleton and reduced calcium secretion in breast milk (Kaska et al., 2013). Calcium absorption increases during pregnancy and additional amounts are not usually required (World Health Organisation, 2013). See chapter 6 for more information about calcium.

Iodine requirements are increased by more than 45% during pregnancy, especially during the first trimester, and half of pregnant woman are iodine deficient. Iodine is needed for development of your baby's brain and nervous system. Maternal iodine deficiency has been associated with increased incidence of miscarriage, stillbirth, and birth defects (Linus Pauling Institute, 2011). There are no specific recommendations for the pregnant woman after bariatric surgery, however Kaska et al., (2013) recommend an intake of 250mcg a day of iodine.

Homocysteine is discussed in chapter 2 and we recommend it is measured prior to conception.

Homocysteine at levels of 15 Imol/tHcy/L or above have been associated with:

- Neural tube defects
- Congenital heart defects
- Recurrent early pregnancy loss
- Abruption of the placenta
- Preeclampsia
- Foetal loss
- Slightly increased chance of babies being born small for gestational age (Hogeveen et al., 2012)

Gastrointestinal screen

From an optimal nutrition perspective we would also recommend a screen for intestinal probiotic bacteria. Unfriendly bacteria contribute to sweet cravings, insulin resistance, obesity (Clemente et al., 2012; Shen et al., 2013), bloating, flatulence (Manichanh et al., 2014) and vaginosis (Mastromarino et al., 2013).

Beneficial bacteria make vitamin B12 and Vitamin K2 and help reduce bloating, abdominal pain and flatulence. There is mounting evidence for the use of probiotics in weight-loss (Delzenne et al., 2011; Sanz et al., 2013; Sanchez et al., 2014). See chapter 3 for more information on gut health.

4.4 Before Pregnancy

Are you entering pregnancy with Polycystic Ovary Syndrome (PCOS), diabetes or hypertension?

Are you morbidly obese?

Obese women are much more likely to experience a

larger number of complications, including spontaneous abortion, gestational diabetes or hypertension, pre-eclampsia, excessive blood loss with caesarean, wound infections or problems with anaesthetics, as well as being more prone to postnatal depression (Dixon et al., 2005; Kaska et al., 2013).

This list can seem quite daunting and if this applies to you then it may be worthwhile finding some support before pregnancy in order to reduce the risk of some of these complications.

4.5 Key recommendations for women following bariatric surgery

- ✓ Reliable contraception for 12 – 24 months after surgery
- ✓ Prenatal Multi-vitamin – 1-a-day to include vitamin A as a natural beta carotene, zinc (15mg) copper (2mg), iodine (100-150mg) and magnesium
- ✓ Folic Acid*** – 400mcg daily – replace with additional doses if deficiency has been confirmed.
- ✓ Vitamin D3 – 400-6,000IU/day depending on status
- ✓ Calcium citrate – 1500mg daily (take 2 hours away from multivitamin)
- ✓ Elemental Iron – 40-65mg/day
- ✓ Vitamin B12 – 350mcg/day orally, replace with additional doses if deficiency has been confirmed.
- ✓ Regular laboratory tests
- ✓ Regular ultrasound scans follow up which evaluates foetal growth and mineralisation of skeleton
- ✓ Close follow up of weight changes during pregnancy and postpartum.
(Kominiarek, 2011; Kaska et al., 2013)

***Around 40% to 60% of the population has genetic polymorphisms that impair the conversion of supplemental folic acid to its active form, L-Methylfolate. It makes sense therefore to supplement with the most bioavailable form (Greenberg & Bell, 2011). The supplement name you are looking for is 5 L-Methyl-tetrahydrofolate or 5 formyl tetrahydrofolate. See chapters 6 and 7.

In general women may swap from their regular multivitamin to a prenatal multivitamin prior to conception. All supplement plans should be modified and personalised after laboratory testing. In the USA only half of women had nutritional evaluations and they were mostly instigated due to anaemia. Increased testing may help identify nutrient deficiencies and prevent consequences for maternal and child health (Gadgil et al., 2014). The importance of this cannot be underestimated.

4.6 What you eat and what it has to do with your baby.

A wide range of factors influences foetal growth and development. A number of these are lifestyle choices that we make, such as smoking, alcohol intake and nutritional intake, where as other factors are essentially fixed at conception (Prentice, 2003).

The uterine environment and maternal health has a central role in foetal programming (Prentice, 2003), which means that what you eat and how you live is literally affecting the genes in your foetus, and in some cases your grandchildren's genes are also affected. The power of food really is incredible.

There is extensive scientific evidence on maternal diet and foetal development. Here are a few interesting studies we wanted to share:

• Xylitol

Pregnant mums who chewed xylitol gum delayed dental cavities in their children measured up to 2 years of age as it reduced a transmission of mutans streptococci (responsible for tooth decay) and reduced dental cavities compared to fluoride by up to 70% at age 5 years (Isokangas et al., 2000).

• Asthma

Pregnant mums who consume higher levels of vitamin D, vitamin E, or/and probiotics help prevent asthma in their infants (Yong et al., 2013).

• Fat and reproductive organs

High fat diet in pregnant mums affects reproductive systems in newborn girls and boys (Papadopoulou et al., 2013).

Maternal diet alters the metabolism of the foetus in later life. Poor maternal diet has been associated with reduced birth weight, increased blood pressure, increased insulin resistance, and increased incidence of type 2 diabetes-mellitus in newborns (Boo & Harding, 2006). These are commonly seen in newborns of mums who are obese or who have recently had bariatric surgery. Some argue, including us, that this could change if you are optimally nourished (Boo & Harding, 2006).

> **Once you are optimally nourished, then you should plan to conceive.**

4.7 How long between surgery and pregnancy?

Recommendations suggest you wait between 12-24 months post-surgery before attempting pregnancy (Armstrong, 2010), with 12 months being the minimum (Khan et al., 2013). This is because, due to the rapid weight-loss you experience and the small amount of food you are able to consume, the foetus may become undernourished. This is all well and good as long as you are aiming to be optimally nourished when you do try to conceive, otherwise you may have only made yourself further malnourished, due to reduced food intake.

There are only a handful of studies about this subject and some groups suggest that measurable outcomes, such as achieving a stabilised weight and correcting nutritional deficiencies, are more appropriate than solely focusing on a specific time period (Alberta Health Care Services, 2012).

Women who had a shorter gap between the weight-loss operation and pregnancy may have a higher rate of miscarriage (Guelinckx et al., 2009). One study found a 31% miscarriage rate among women who became pregnant within 18 months of their surgeries, compared to 18% miscarriage rate in women who became pregnant after 18 months (Khan et al., 2013). The closer to surgery the higher the chances of reduced foetal growth and labour tends to be induced more often when pregnancy occurs closer to surgery than for those who waited for a longer time period (Guelinckx et al., 2009). The research is conflicting and this may be due to the wide range of factors involved in pregnancy as mentioned at the start of this chapter. Band adjustments are more likely to be needed if pregnancy occurs close to having a band fitted (Haward et al., 2011) and close surveillance of maternal weight and nutritional status is advisable, particularly if conception occurs within the first year after surgery (Alatishe et al., 2012).

4.8 Food and Pregnancy

At the time of going to print we were unable to find any guidelines for active band management during pregnancy. A 2014 review by Chilelli et al., say, *"screening for nutritional complications, such as micro and macronutrient deficiencies, has been very little explored in the literature. Only one study assessed the differences before and after pregnancy in women who had previously undergone bariatric surgery"* and this study was based on RYGB, not banding, so may or may not be relevant.

The Journal of Women's Health has also recently (2014) published a paper calling for practice guidelines due to the higher risk of nutrient deficiencies (Maggard-Gibbons, 2014).

Some things to consider are:

Your needs are individual, if you have not had a vitamin and mineral screen carried out, we strongly recommend having one. Adapt your food and nutrient intake according to your results.

You are NOT eating for two! However you should be optimally nourished not only for you but also for your growing baby.

Water. It may be hard to consume the extra water your body needs throughout pregnancy therefore dehydration could become an issue. Take water with you everywhere and sip continuously through the day, add vegetable juices and soups to your diet, and increase the amount of foods that have high water content into your diet, such as cucumbers and watermelons.

Ensure you have adequate protein. The need for protein increases as your pregnancy develops. It is required for growth of the foetus, placenta and for the changes that occur within your body including after the birth and breast-feeding. The UK government recommends a normal weight pregnant woman increases their protein intake by around 13% or 6g a day, this is to a total of around 52g a day (Williamson, 2006). For pregnant bariatric patients the minimum amount recommended is 60g per day (Kominiarek, 2011). You may require good quality protein powders to meet this intake.

Include healthy fats such as oily fish, maximum two portions a week, ground nuts and seeds, or nut butters, avocados and oils including olive, walnut, hemp and flaxseed. These are needed for the development of your baby's brain and nervous system. They are also essential for keeping a balanced mood and to maintain supple skin.

Include beans and lentils for fibre. Constipation is common in pregnancy and these fibres help maintain regular bowel movements and clear toxins from the body.

Vegetables, fruits and whole grains provide a wide range of vitamins and minerals as well as fibre.

Zinc levels decrease by around 30% in 'normal' pregnancies and levels could be even lower after having weight-loss surgery (Kaska et al., 2013).

Only 15% of pregnant women have adequate choline intake (Lynch, 2015). Choline is found in seafood, eggs, chicken, and green leafy vegetables.

Avoid alcohol, caffeine, sugar and white refined foods.

Please speak with your health care provider or visit The

Foods Standards Agency (UK) website for the most up-to-date list of high-risk foods and drinks to avoid during pregnancy.

Summary sheet of foods to avoid whilst pregnant

Avoid these foods	Why	What to do instead
Soft CHEESES made from unpasteurized milk, including Brie, feta, Camembert, Roquefort, Queso fresco	May contain *E. coli* or *Listeria*.	Eat hard cheeses, such as cheddar or Swiss cheese. Check the label and make sure that the cheese is made from pasteurized milk
Certain kinds of FISH, such as shark, swordfish, king mackerel and tuna.	Contains high levels of mercury that may harm your baby's nervous system.	Eat up to 12 ounces a week of fish and shellfish that are lower in mercury, such as shrimp, salmon, pollock, and catfish.
Unpasteurized MILK	May contain bacteria such as *Campylobacter, E. coli, Listeria,* or *Salmonella.*	Drink pasteurized milk. Or use alternatives such as nut, rice or quinoa milk.
Raw SHELLFISH, such as oysters and clams, MEAT and POULTRY	May contain *Vibrio* bacteria.	Cook shellfish to 145° F. Cook meat thoroughly.
Raw or undercooked SPROUTS, such as alfalfa, clover, mung bean, and radish	May contain *E. coli* or *Salmonella.*	Only use fresh sprouts. If they have slight browning, discard.
UNWASHED fruits and vegetables	Taxoplasmosis, which may damage your baby.	Wash your fruits and vegetables thoroughly
Deli TURKEY	May contain *Listeria*	

Adapted from: U.S. Department of Health & Human Services, Foods Standards Agency, UK, Oster (2013).

4.9 What Else?

4.9.1 Nausea and Vomiting

This may be worse for you in early pregnancy; you may need to have your band loosened. Balancing your blood sugar by including protein (yogurt, eggs, or protein powder based smoothies) with your meals may help.

Ginger may also help calm your stomach and relieve sickness. Fresh ginger can be peeled, thinly sliced and eaten raw, or add slices of peeled raw ginger to hot water (and lemon if desired) and drink as a tea.

4.9.2 Weight Gain

A natural process of pregnancy, this needs to be discussed with your health professional in order to keep it under control. The Institute of Medicine Guidelines recommends that women who are overweight (BMI 25-29.9) gain between 15-25lbs, and women who are obese (all classes BMI 30+) gain between 11-20lbs. According to the American College of Obstetrics and Gynecologists (2013) there should be some differentiation between classes of obesity in women as this weight gain may be too high for some. Personalised care and advice is recommended (ACOG, 2013).

Studies show women with gastric bands gain less weight, have lower rates of pre-eclampsia, gestational diabetes, and hypertension than those who are obese without a band. However, this is still higher than those who are overweight or of a normal weight (Bar-Zohar et al., 2006; Ducarme et al., 2007; Maggard et al., 2008).

4.9.3 Hernias

Some surgeons will deflate the band totally in order to prevent hernias at around 36 weeks, this also allows for you to optimise nutrition prior to lactation.

4.9.4 Band Mechanics in Pregnancy

Bands migrate in up to 29% of reported cases during pregnancy bands migrate, resulting in vomiting, severe dehydration, electrolyte disturbances and band leakage (Guelinckx et al., 2009).

5.0 Band Loosened or Not?

A 2013 Cochrane Review by Jefferys and colleagues found that no conclusion could currently be drawn regarding best management of the band in pregnancy due to a lack of evidence and wide variations of management in clinical settings. Pilone and colleagues small study (2014) recommended loosening bands in symptomatic patients only.

However, just as we were going to print Cornthwaite et al., (2015) published data saying that bands should not be inflated *throughout pregnancy*, as it is detrimental to the foetus. The optimum timing of band adjustment is unknown. A personalised approach remains the best method for patient management.

Bands should not be inflated throughout pregnancy.

Cornthwaite et al., 2015

Considerations when making a decision:

- Stage in pregnancy?
- How well nourished are you at the start of your pregnancy?
- How well nourished are you throughout each trimester?
- What is your weight at the start of pregnancy?
- What is your weight through each trimester?
- Do you have nausea and vomiting?
- How is the band feeling?
- How is your baby growing and developing?
- Do you have any pregnancy complications?

Advantages of the band being inflated:

- Limit food intake
- Limit weight gain
- Might help reduce high blood pressure
- Might help reduce diabetes
- Might help with outcomes for mother and baby

Disadvantages of the band being inflated:

- Less nutrient intake for mother and baby
- Band complications such as:
  - Nausea
  - Vomiting
  - Band slippage
  - Hernias
  - Increased intra-abdominal pressure

6.0 What About Contraception?

As patients are advised to avoid pregnancy in the first 1-2 years after surgery to coincide with the most weight-loss, contraception is an important consideration.

Scientific studies are sparse and conflicting.

Obese women are less likely to use contraception than normal weight women (Chuang et al., 2005) and those that do use it, are not always using the most effective form (Chin et al., 2009).

There are concerns about the efficacy of the oral contraceptive in obese women and in those after bariatric surgery. Suggestions have been proposed for recommendations to be made to have local delivery of hormones as by the vaginal ring, or an IUD.

It is worth bearing in mind that people who work with family planning professionals are more successful at preventing unplanned pregnancy than those who don't.

The Family Planning Association has a really useful contraceptive tool on its website.

We recommend you use the longer length questionnaire to assess your contraceptive needs and choices as this includes data and success rates for a range of BMIs.

http://www.fpa.org.uk/contraception-help/my-contraception-tool

Summary:

- ✓ A wide range of factors are involved in preconception, fertility and pregnancy

- ✓ Neither men nor women should have weight-loss surgery solely to increase chances of fertility

- ✓ In men sperm parameters should be tested prior to conceiving

- ✓ Sexual satisfaction improves in men and women after surgery

- ✓ Banding is safe for mum and newborn

- ✓ Get pre-conception biochemical and functional tests

- ✓ Wait 12-24 months after surgery before conceiving

- ✓ Be optimally nourished

- ✓ What you eat affects your baby

- ✓ Have a supportive team working with you

- ✓ Preconception supplements

- ✓ Consider your personalised nutrient requirements for pregnancy

- ✓ Regular ultrasound scans

- ✓ Discuss and decide upon contraception

Chapter 5

Food & Drink

A new way of life, not a diet.

5.1 Food

Eating and drinking should be an enjoyable experience; however what you eat or drink has a huge impact on your health, mood and weight. Diets and yo-yo dieting is not what we advocate. We are here to encourage eating, as eating is one of life's pleasures, but eating to fuel your body, your mind and giving you the nutrients you need to be healthy.

What is refined?

Simply put, refined food has been to a factory and processed in some form or another. Maybe it has been changed from a wholegrain (like brown rice) to a shiny white grain (white rice), during this process many of the nutrients are stripped out and we are left with the energy part of the food, not the nutritional part. Biscuits, cookies, cakes, chewy bars, chocolate, crisps, crackers, many breakfast cereals, pasta and bread, to name a few, have been refined.

And unrefined?

If it grows in nature, such as fruits, vegetables, roots and leaves, nuts, seeds, beans and lentils, or lives naturally, such as animals, birds, fish and some of their by-products, such as eggs, then it's not refined and much better for you.

Refined foods, such as white bread and rice, and stimulants such as chocolate, tea and coffee, release glucose quickly into the bloodstream. The burst of energy these foods provide is short-lived as the body will promptly release insulin in order to lower blood sugar levels. As the blood sugar level drops, the subsequent energy low leaves you reaching for the chocolate or coffee – thereby promoting the rollercoaster of energy highs and lows associated with blood sugar imbalance (also known as dysglycemia). This is linked with mood swings, headaches, dizziness, weight gain, pre-menstrual tension and could eventually lead to insulin resistance.

To help control blood sugar levels, eat regularly – aim for three meals each day and if you are hungry then a small healthy snack mid-morning or afternoon. When blood sugar is being easily maintained you should reduce the snacks until you are eating just three meals a day.

✓ Eating high quality protein with every meal and snack helps slow digestion, which slows the release of glucose from the food in to the bloodstream.

✓ Choose brown rice and whole meal bread (if you are able to eat bread) and include lentils, pulses and plenty of vegetables in your daily meals. They are rich in fibre, which helps maintain blood sugar balance.

✓ Increase the amount of oily fish, nuts and seeds you eat – they provide essential fatty acids which may help to prevent insulin resistance. Fish is fantastic for gastric band wearers as it is high in protein and easier to chew and digest than meat. Nuts and seeds may need to be ground.

5.2 Drink

What you drink is just as important as what you eat, and for some people even more important.

Sugar and Artificially Sweetened Drinks (soft drinks)

If you drink these, reduce and then omit them from your diet. If you decided you only ever wanted to make one change to your diet – make it this one. They have absolutely no benefit to health whatsoever.

There is a dose-response relationship between soft drinks and weight gain; the more you drink the more weight you gain (Hu, 2013). Evidence clearly demonstrates that these common drinks not only contribute to obesity, but also diabetes, cardiovascular disease and more (Grimes et al., 2013; Hu & Malik, 2010; Malik et al., 2011; Malik et al., 2013). After drinking high fructose corn syrup, in soft drinks, triglyceride markers that contribute to cardiovascular disease were increased in just two weeks (Stanhope et al., 2015); imagine what is happening to your waistline and your heart if you drink this every day.

Weighing up the evidence.

A 2013 review concluded that industry bias may be affecting conclusions with regards to sugar sweetened beverages and weight gain or obesity, with those funded by industry being five times more likely to find no association than those that were independently funded (Bes-Restrollo et al., 2013).

In general we don't recommend carbonated beverages, as you may have guessed. However, sparkling water may be used to help dislodge food that gets trapped in your band.

Water

Our bodies consist of around 60% water with fat tissue having less than lean tissue. Water is required for our brain to make hormones and neurotransmitters, lubrication and cushioning of joints, spine, and other sensitive areas, to maintain our temperature, and to aid excretion of waste through urination, sweat, and bowel movements. People often tell us in clinic that they don't like the taste of water, if this is also how you feel then we recommend trying different bottled water and see which taste you do prefer. The more you do it, the easier it will become to drink, as your taste buds adapt. Alternatively you can make your own flavoured water.

Making Your Own Flavoured Water

Easily add more taste and nutrients to your water by adding slices of fruit, veg, herbs or spices. Here are some of our favourites:

- Cucumber and mint leaves

- Strawberry, apple and mint

- Slices of lemon, orange or grapefruit with sliced fresh ginger

- Chunks of apple, pear or a few berries

- Orange and cinnamon

- Lime and ginger

Tea and Coffee

If you are drinking tea and coffee try alternatives such as herbal teas, which have many varied benefits, and swapping your coffee to dandelion, chicory (both of which support liver function) or barley. People who have one or less caffeinated drinks are more successful with their weight-loss post-bariatric surgery than those who consume more than one cup a day (Safer et al., 2013).

Green tea is one exception as it has a number of health benefits, including reducing blood pressure, total cholesterol and LDL cholesterol (Onakpoya et al., 2014), as well as reducing fasting insulin and having a positive effect on insulin resistance (Mozaffari-Khosravi et al., 2014). A Cochrane Review (2012) showed that participants had a small but not significant weight-loss (0.2kg – 3.5kg compared to the control group). This small weight-loss can mean a lot to some people therefore we recommend green tea to our clients.

Coconut Water

We like coconut water because it's not only delicious but it's also good for you. Coconut water contains minerals (especially sodium, potassium, magnesium and calcium) so can be used to effectively rehydrate the body by replenishing electrolytes. It also contains B vitamins, vitamin C, amino acids and a number of antioxidants (Yong et al., 2009).

Milk

There is conflicting information on milk and dairy products for obesity and weight management, which is due to differences in the type, quantity, quality and fortification of dairy product being evaluated. The dietary assessment and length of studies vary, as does the age of the participant. A 2011 systematic review concluded that there is insufficient evidence that dairy intake is associated with weight status (Louie et al., 2011).

Putting weight management aside, humans have no nutritional requirement for animal milk and many populations consume little, if any, milk due to cultural preferences, lack of availability, or due to a lactase deficiency (Ludwig & Willett, 2013). The Physicians Committee for Responsible Medicine (2014) highlights the detrimental effects of milk with regards to a number of serious health conditions and report that milk consumption increases our intake of synthetic hormones, pesticides and antibiotics.

Studies funded by the dairy industry (along with sugar-sweetened beverages and fruit juice studies) are eight times more likely to show overall positive effects than more independently funded studies (Lesser et al., 2007). No wonder there are so many mixed messages.

We recommend:

Trying alternative sources of milk such as organic almond, cashew, Brazil, quinoa and rice milks. If you want to drink cow's milk then choosing unsweetened, organic options makes most sense. If you are worried about your calcium intake go to Chapter 6 – Nutrients to find other good sources.

Alcohol

Alcohol varies widely in nutrient content and the dose at which it causes more harm than good is highly variable and depends on genetic variations. Potential harm has been associated, even at recommended intake levels, and should be avoided by those with liver disease or history of alcoholism (Katz, 2008).

A retrospective study took data from over 11,000 patients who had undergone different types of bariatric surgery between 1980 and 2006 in Sweden. They found that patients who had undergone gastric bypass had more than double the risk of alcohol abuse compared to patients who had gastric bands (Ostlund et al., 2013). Another study earlier in 2013 found similar results and concluded that banding showed no difference to controls (Svensson et al., 2013).

> **If you are partial to a weekend tipple, make sure it's small.**

Aloe Vera

Aloe Vera juice has quite a distinct taste, and only a small amount is needed (a shot glass will probably suffice). You'll notice we have included it in the early stages of the meal plan as it has anti-inflammatory properties, helps with wound healing, helps balance insulin response (so may help reduce sugar cravings) and has antibacterial and anti-viral properties. It also works as a laxative. We recommend buying the aloe juice sold in glass bottles, rather than the plastic ones, and it's available at good quality health food stores.

In summary, choose water as your first option, forget the sugar-laden or artificially sweetened carbonated soft drinks – and if you are partial to weekend tipple, make sure it's small.

5.3 Food Quality

The quality of your food and drink is hugely important. It is the information that directly washes over your cells and your genes every time you consume anything, every day of the week, every week of the year. A diet that is based around natural whole-foods and plants, and that is low in processed foods, has been proven time and again to reduce obesity, type 2 diabetes, cardiovascular disease, high blood pressure and more (Hu & Willett, 2002; Liu et al., 2003; Craig & Mangels 2009; Grant, 2012; Tuso et al., 2013; Katz & Mellor, 2014; Sala-Vila et al., 2015; Turner, McGrievy et al., 2015). Convenience foods may save time in the short-term but longer-term negatively impact your health. Food additives found in common convenience foods promote obesity, adapt gut flora, and lead to metabolic syndrome (which leads to type 2 diabetes) (Chassaing et al., 2015).

5.4 Mindful Eating

There are a number of books written on the importance of mindful eating and those who eat more mindfully are more successful with their weight-loss five years and more, post-bariatric surgery, than those who eat mindlessly (Safer et al., 2013).

The Center for Mindful Eating recommends you:

• Allow yourself to become aware of the positive and nurturing opportunities available through food selection and preparation by respecting your own inner wisdom.

- Use all your senses to choose to eat food that is both satisfying to you and nourishing to your body.

- Acknowledge your responses to food (likes, dislikes or neutral) without judgement.

- Become aware of physical hunger and satiety cues to guide your decisions to start and stop eating.

Digestion begins in the mouth and good digestion is essential to enable you to absorb the nutrients from your food, therefore our advice is that you:

- Be present – sit and eat at a table, ban phones, TV's and computers from meal times, be aware of what you are eating and savour it.
- Eat in a relaxed state.
- Eat slowly – putting your knife, fork or spoon down between mouthfuls may help.
- Chew thoroughly – count the number of times you chew each mouthful to slow you down if need be.
- Listen to your body – are you still hungry or have you had enough to eat?
- Why are you eating – are you hungry or are you upset, anxious, angry or happy?

Obesity reduces chewing function. Chewing food activates histamine fibres that trigger satiety, reduces visceral fat, increases the absorption of nutrients and enhances digestive motility. Having your mouth, chewing motion, and teeth checked is recommended prior to surgery.

Veyrune et al., 2008

5.5 A New Way of Life, Not a Diet

This is not a diet – we all know diets don't work in the long-term. The ideas and recommendations are aimed at providing you with the nutritious foods you need for as long as you wear a band.

The following is general information and our suggestions for a post-operative eating plan. Your speed of recovery from the operation and your ability to eat varies from one individual to another so rather than give time limits we have suggested eating phases and that you move from one phase to another as and when you feel ready.

On the day of the operation you will be sipping water only. By Day 2 you will have moved on to Phase 1.

5.5.1 Phase 1: Free Fluids

This phase is likely to last a couple of days or up to a week depending on how you feel. Once you are taking fluids easily you can move on to Phase 2.

Meal Ideas: Phase 1 – Free Fluids

Plain water (not carbonated)
Coconut water
Herbal teas
Diluted fruit or vegetable juice
Milk

Why are you saying having a juice, not a smoothie?

Juicing fruits is not the healthiest way to eat fruit due to the high sugar content once the pulp has been removed. However, we recommend juicing fruits and vegetables during the free fluid stage as this helps give direct nutrients to the body, supports cleansing, healing and energy. Once you have moved on from this stage then we generally recommend smoothies, and particularly encourage reducing or omitting the fruit and increasing the green leaves, vegetables and herbs.

5.5.2 Sample Meal Plan – Phase 1 - Free Fluids

These are just suggestions, please feel free to adapt to suit your taste. This phase is only likely to last a couple of days however a few more have been provided just in case you really are not that hungry or do not feel ready to eat pureed foods yet. We have included calming and healing herb teas such as liquorice, fennel, chamomile and mint as well as aloe vera juice to aid in your recovery from surgery.

Meal	Day 1	Day 2	Day 3	Day 4	Day 5	Day 6	Day 7
Breakfast	Water AND Tea, Herbal or Green Tea or Coffee (inc. dandelion or chicory)	Water AND Tea, Herbal or Green Tea or Coffee (inc. dandelion or chicory)	Water AND Tea, Herbal or Green Tea or Coffee (inc. dandelion or chicory)	Water AND Tea, Herbal or Green Tea or Coffee (inc. dandelion or chicory)	Water AND Tea, Herbal or Green Tea or Coffee (inc. dandelion or chicory)	Water AND Tea, Herbal or Green Tea or Coffee (inc. dandelion or chicory)	Water AND Tea, Herbal or Green Tea or Coffee (inc. dandelion or chicory)
Snack	Glass coconut water, herbal tea or fresh juice	Glass coconut water, fresh juice or herbal tea	Glass coconut water, herbal tea or fresh juice	Glass coconut water, fresh juice or herbal tea	Glass coconut water, herbal tea or fresh juice	Glass coconut water, fresh juice or herbal tea	Glass coconut water, herbal tea or fresh juice
Lunch	Fresh Juice (Berry Blast) and Coconut water	Fresh Juice (Alkalising Juice) and Aloe vera juice	Fresh Juice (Fat Busting Juice) and Coconut water	Fresh Juice (Beet It Juice) and Aloe vera juice	Fresh Juice (Pineapple Green Juice) and Coconut water	Fresh Juice (Cleansing Juice) and Aloe vera juice	Fresh Juice (Green Juice) and Coconut water
Snack	Glass coconut water, fresh juice or herbal tea	Glass coconut water, herbal tea or fresh juice	Glass coconut water, fresh juice or herbal tea	Glass coconut water, herbal tea or fresh juice	Glass coconut water, fresh juice or herbal tea	Glass coconut water, herbal tea or fresh juice	Glass coconut water, fresh juice or herbal tea
Dinner	Vegetable broth and Fennel tea	Bone broth and Peppermint tea	Veg broth and Chamomile tea	Bone broth and Fennel tea	Vegetable broth and Licorice tea	Bone broth and Peppermint tea	Vegetable broth and Chamomile tea

5.5.3 Phase 2: Pureed Food

For the first four weeks or so after having your surgery all food should be pureed and eaten in small quantities so that you're having 4 or 5 small meals each day. The purees should be smooth – a food processor or hand-held blender will do this easily or you could use a potato masher for soft-cooked vegetables. Extra fluid may need to be added to get the puree to the right consistency. Use the cooking water from the vegetables for extra nutrients for savoury foods or diluted fruit juice or water for fruit purees.

The size of each meal should be around 100g/5-6 tablespoons. It is important to eat slowly and take small mouthfuls, and stop eating as soon as you begin to feel full (if you carry on eating at this point you're more likely to vomit).

Do not drink whilst eating but try to drink between 1.5-2 litres (2 1/2 pints) of water every day between meals. Sipping frequently will be easier than trying to down a glassful at a time.

After about 4 weeks you may no longer need to puree to a smooth consistency but still keep food fairly soft and same quantities but with lumps.

After the first band fill, you will feel the band's restriction although it may require a couple of visits to get the band at the right tightness for you. As the pouch is at the top of your stomach, your feeling of fullness may feel more like a tightness or heaviness in your chest.

Meal Ideas: Phase 2 – Pureed Food

Breakfast:
Power-packed smoothie – see Recipes section
Live natural low fat yogurt with some mashed banana or pureed berries
3 tbsp porridge with fruit puree

Lunch/Supper:
Pureed soup – see Recipes for some super nutritious delicious soups

Snacks: – 1 a day between meals
Stewed apple
Mashed banana
Live natural low fat yogurt with pureed fruit

Drinks:
Plain water (not carbonated)
Coconut water
Herbal tea
Diluted fruit or vegetable juice

5.5.4 Sample Meal Plan – Phase 2 – Pureed Foods

This plan is just to give you an idea of what to eat and when – please feel free to change the smoothie or soup listed.

For the first four weeks after having your gastric band fitted all food should be pureed and eaten in small quantities so that you're having 4 or 5 small meals each day. The purees should be smooth – a food processor or hand-held blender will do this easily.

WEEKLY MEAL PLAN

Meal	Day 1	Day 2	Day 3	Day 4	Day 5	Day 6	Day 7
Breakfast	Berry smoothie or 3 tbsp porridge with berry puree	Live plain low fat yogurt with pureed apple and cinnamon	Avocado smoothie	Green smoothie	3 tbsp porridge with pear and ginger puree	Live plain low fat yogurt with pureed apple and cinnamon.	Green smoothie
Mid morning	Small cup Vegetable juice/broth	Small bowl of stewed pear	Mashed banana	Live natural low fat yogurt with fruit puree	Small bowl of stewed apple with cinnamon	Small cup of soup or bone broth	Mashed avocado, olive oil & lemon
Lunch	Pumpkin & Lentil soup	Chickpea and leek soup	Beetroot Buzz smoothie	Roasted Mushroom soup	Watercress and Butter Bean soup	Spicy Watercress & Broccoli soup.	Chickpea and Leek soup
Mid afternoon	Small glass of smoothie	Mashed avocado, olive oil & lemon	Small bowl of stewed apple	Small glass of smoothie	Cup of soup or bone broth	Mashed banana	Small bowl of stewed pear
Dinner	Watercress and Butter Bean soup and Ginger and lemon tea	Pumpkin and Lentil soup and Fennel tea	Vegetable soup and Chamomile tea	Easy Peasy Green soup and Licorice and fennel tea	Vegetable soup and Redbush (Rooiboos) tea	Roasted Mushroom Soup and Peppermint tea	Carrot, Coriander & Lentil soup and Ginger and lemon tea

Remember to make soups in large batches and freeze them in the portion size you need... then you have an 'instant', nutritious and delicious lunch or supper to hand. After a few weeks you will be able to make the soups lumpier. There are recipes for more non-liquidised soups in the Recipes section.

It is vital to eat slowly, chew well and pause between each mouthful. Eat small meals at regular intervals. When you're ready, which could be another few weeks, move on to Phase 3: Proper meals.

5.5.5 Phase 3: Proper Meals

Real solid food! Now you can begin the food plan you'll follow for the foreseeable future... maybe the rest of your life.

What you are able to eat will differ between individuals but the most important thing is to eat for optimum nutrition, not only weight-loss but for your long-term health and wellbeing.

The amount you can eat is highly individual – you're probably looking at somewhere between a golf ball and a tennis ball size serving but you will become the expert on your new stomach. You don't want to stretch the pouch so take time to listen to your body and learn to trust yourself.

Meal Ideas: Phase 3 – Proper Meals

Breakfast:
Power-packed smoothie – see Recipes
Porridge with berries and ground seeds
Natural low fat or 0% yogurt with berries, nuts, and seeds
Scrambled egg

Lunch:
Soup – the variety is endless – see Recipes
Hummus with crudité
Omelette with herbs
Falafel and Tasty Carrot salad – see Recipes

Dinner: see Recipes for these and many more tasty suppers
Chicken and lentil curry
Cod, chorizo and chickpea stew
Salmon with soy, ginger & spring onion
Turkey burger

Snacks: – check out our Recipes for other healthy snack ideas
Small pot natural yogurt with handful nuts
Crudité sticks with nut butter
Piece fruit with handful mixed raw nuts or seeds

Drinks:
Plain water (avoid carbonated)
Coconut water
Herbal tea
Diluted fruit or vegetable juice

5.5.6 Sample Meal Plan – Phase 3 - Proper Meals

Now you can begin the food plan you'll follow for the foreseeable future... maybe the rest of your life.

You will see on the Sample Meal Plan that we have reduced the snack to one a day and ideally you would reduce this so you are eating just three regular meals a day.

These are just suggestions, please feel free to adapt to suit your taste. What you are able to eat will differ between individuals but the most important thing is to eat for your long term health and wellbeing.

Meal	Day 1	Day 2	Day 3	Day 4	Day 5	Day 6	Day 7
Breakfast	Scrambled egg with finely chopped vegetables	Power packed smoothie	Warm and wholesome apple/cinnamon porridge	Protein packed breakfast	Apple, almond & cinnamon pancakes	Omelette with choice of filling	Protein packed breakfast
Lunch	Moroccan spiced soup	Tomato, Carrot and Lentil soup	Omelette with herb salad	Spicy hummus with choice of crudité	Thai style Lentil and Coconut soup	Mediterranean style soup	Scrambled egg with chives
Snack (if necessary)	Small handful seeds and piece of fresh fruit	Natural plain low fat yogurt with ground seeds and fruit puree	Tablespoon hummus with raw veg	Super-Quick Courgette salad	Tablespoon nut butter on an oatcake	Tasty Carrot salad	½ avocado with lemon juice & pepper
Dinner	Cod, chorizo and chickpea stew	Sesame grilled chicken with celeriac mash	Chicken and lentil curry	Salmon with soy, ginger & spring onion	Moroccan chicken with apricots and lemon	Roast fish with herbs and tomatoes	Speedy Hunters Chicken

Band fills and adjustments:

After each band fill, you may need to go back to Phase 1 (Free fluids), progress through Phase 2 (Pureed foods) and on to Phase 3 (Proper meals), as you feel able.

This part is IMPORTANT!

- Eat three healthy, nutritious meals and perhaps one snack each day. Don't skip a meal and don't graze through the day.
- Eat a source of protein with each meal (i.e. plain yogurt, seeds, nuts, lentils, meat, fish). Protein is not only essential for the body's maintenance and repair, it also takes time to eat and digest, keeping you feeling fuller for longer.
- Include fruit or vegetables with every meal, for fibre as well as their many other vital nutrients.
- Fat is important! – The essential fatty acids found in oily fish (i.e. salmon, mackerel, sardines) and nuts/seeds not only support energy metabolism but also help burn excess stored fat so encourages weight-loss.
- Carbohydrates such as bread, pasta and rice may be more difficult to eat. Choose unrefined, whole grain for extra fibre and B vitamins to support energy.

Watch out for...

- Sauce, cream or mayonnaise with meals – they may make it easier to eat but will have a big impact on the calories consumed.
- Drinking your calories – avoid caffeine, alcohol, milkshakes, carbonated drinks and undiluted fruit juice.
- Sugar and fat – to make food palatable manufacturers use sugar, fat or both. If something is 'low fat' be wary

of how much sugar it has. It would be better to have the 'full fat' low sugar variety.

Top tips!
- Change to a small plate or bowl
- Eat with a teaspoon or children's cutlery
- Take small mouthfuls
- Eat slowly and chew well

5.6 Top 20 Foods for Gastric Band Wearers

We have discovered that it is very hard for us to choose favourite foods and this list could actually go on for some time! There are so many wonderful foods out there, so take this as a starting tool, not a prescription. However, here are our top twenty, chosen according to these criteria.

Criteria:
- ✓ Easy to consume and digest
- ✓ High nutrient quantity
- ✓ High water content
- ✓ Won't get stuck in the band
- ✓ Healing for digestive tract
- ✓ Reduce symptoms common in gastric band wearers (dehydration, bloating, gut flora, inflammation)
- ✓ Rich in iron, vitamins A, D, E and K and antioxidants
- ✓ Fruits and vegetables that contain anti-obesity properties

1. Oily fish

Oily fish such as salmon, mackerel, sardines, pilchards, trout, herring and fresh tuna are great sources of lean protein as well as anti-inflammatory essential fatty acids. Although white fish also contain essential fats, they have much less than oily fish.

2. Chickpeas/lentils/beans

Great sources of vegetable protein and the all-important fibre that will help to keep your bowels working well. Pulses are also good sources of prebiotics, the food that keeps your gut bacteria happy.

3. Chicory and watercress

The Egyptians used chicory as early as 5,000 years ago as a medicinal food. The most commonly studied use of chicory for a health complaint is for chronic hepatitis, however it is also used historically for constipation, diabetes, for gastrointestinal disorders, and weight-loss and obesity. The thick roots are sometimes used as a coffee substitute and they help support liver detoxification (Natural Standards Database, 2014). Use in salads or as an edible garnish.

Watercress is rich in iodine that help stimulates the thyroid, purify the blood, relieve phlegm and may break up kidney and bladder stones. It can be difficult for some band wearers to eat raw. If this is your experience we suggest you make soup with it.

Note: Make sure you thoroughly wash your watercress under running clean water.

4. Red onions

These little beauties are rich in quercitin, anthocyanins and thiosulphinates. These compounds have been found to inhibit fat cell growth, reduce inflammation in obese body tissue and reduce blood glucose levels. The outer layers contain more than the inner layers and you can lose around 15% of the compounds by boiling them for just five minutes. It appears the compounds might be lost due to heat degradation but it may be that they are also water-soluble (Williams et al., 2013). For now if you want them cooked then it seems best to quickly steam or stir-fry them. You could also add them raw to tomato-based vegetable juices or raw tomato soups.

5. Leeks

The medicinal value of leeks has been valued for thousands of years and the green leaf contains more powerful antioxidant properties than the white shaft (Bernaert et al., 2012). Perfect cleansing food that also acts as a diuretic. Eliminates uric acid in gout. Contains potassium, vitamin K, calcium, folate and vitamin A.

6. Mushrooms

Mushrooms support many systems of the body including cardiovascular health and immune function. They contain calcium, iron, magnesium, vitamin B1, B2 (Furlani & Godoy, 2008), B3, B5, folate and zinc. Brown and white mushrooms have high amounts of vitamin A, Shiitake have high amounts of B1 and B5 and Portobello have high amounts of B2 and B3 (Gaglarirmak, 2011).

Mushrooms also contain beta-glucans; these promote specific responses to the immune system protecting the body from allergic reactions and have powerful anti-inflammatory effects. The beta glucans found in mushrooms also support the metabolism of fats in the human body and contributes to weight-loss (Rop et al., 2009). This is supported by a recent study that showed swapping red meat for mushrooms enhanced weight-loss, weight maintenance and health parameters (Poddar et al., 2013).

We recommend including a wide variety of mushrooms to your diet including brown, white, button, oyster, shiitake and reishi.

White mushrooms have high levels of the antioxidant ergothioneine, which protects against cardiovascular disease.

Reishi mushrooms thin the blood, lower blood sugar levels, act as an anti-inflammatory agent and may help reduce allergies, and support sleep patterns and liver function.

Shiitake mushrooms help control cholesterol, improve immune responses, act as an antiviral agent, and fresh shiitake is a source of vitamin D2 (Natural Standards, 2014; Powell, 2013).

7. Broccoli

Is an excellent source of fibre that also helps stimulate the liver, aiding detoxification. It lowers LDL (the bad) cholesterol in people with high cholesterol and is a perfect fat fighting food. The compounds in broccoli are being studied as a functional food for weight-loss. While they are trying to work out how to do that, it's probably quicker and easier to eat the broccoli itself. Broccoli contains more than 80 micronutrients and is high in B vitamins, vitamin C, folate, calcium and magnesium (Natural Standards, 2014).

8. Red, blue and black berries

Fresh **raspberries** support weight-loss due to the fact they are low in calories, have a low glycaemic load and are high in fibre. They are full of vitamin C, B3, magnesium, phosphorus and potassium, and ½ cup contains 4g fibre.

Strawberries have antiviral, antibacterial and anti-inflammatory properties. They contain vitamin A, vitamin C, vitamin K, beta-carotene and folate. Strawberries aid iron absorption due to their vitamin C content (Natural Standards Database, 2014).

Blueberries may be used as a natural laxative. They help cleanse the blood and improve circulation.

Blackberries are a great tonic food, a good blood cleanser and used to relieve diarrhoea. They contain magnesium, potassium, phosphorus, beta-carotene and vitamin C.

Note: Raspberry ketones are the compound that gives red raspberries their lovely aroma. They are extracted from the fruit and sold as a weight-loss supplement. We recommend using whole natural foods as much as possible and until there is further clinical evidence do not currently recommend using raspberry ketones to our clients.

9. Apples

There are more than 7,500 types of apples, so if you think you don't like apples try another type – you have plenty more to choose from.

Apples are used to relieve allergies, constipation, diarrhoea, support management of diabetes, and boost levels of friendly bacteria in the gut. They help reduce total cholesterol and are well known for supporting toxin excretion (Natural Standards, 2014).

Apples are good for the teeth and do not promote cariogenic bacteria. Apples contain pectin, quercetin, calcium, magnesium, vitamin C and beta-carotene. **Pectin** is broken down and used as fuel by our gut microbes. **Quercetin** has been shown to have anti-inflammatory effects in the body (Hamalainen et al., 2007) and inhibits the growth of fat cells, and reduces markers of inflammation and insulin resistance in human fat cells (Williams et al., 2013).

Apple puree makes a great sweetener and is commonly used as a binding ingredient in homemade snack bars and muffins.

Note: Apple juice may not be a good choice pre-operatively, as it increases gastric volume and pH as well as feelings of irritability, thirst and hunger in some people (Natural Standards, 2014).

10. Garlic

Garlic is one of the most researched medicinal foods and is a powerful antibacterial, antiviral, anti parasitic, and antifungal agent.

Traditionally it has been used to treat infection, colds, diabetes, heart disease, warts, bladder disorders, fatigue, hormonal disorders and much more (Natural Standards Database, 2014). Clinically, garlic is predominantly used for lowering blood pressure, cholesterol, and glucose concentration, as well as for the prevention of arteriosclerosis and cancer (Tsai et al., 2012).

Evidence shows garlic is beneficial for a wide range of health issues associated with being obese such as hyperlipidaemia, hypertension, cardiovascular disease risk, circulation, angina, common colds, Helicobacter pylori infection, dental conditions, hepatitis and heavy metal/lead toxicity (Natural Standards Database, 2014).

11. Cucumbers

In India cucumbers are traditionally used for headaches, and the juice used to reduce acne (Kumar et al., 2010). In Europe they are well known for their cleansing and diuretic properties. Properties in cucumbers help dissolve uric acid that causes kidney and bladder stones as well as helping digestion and regulating blood pressure. Studies also show cucumbers have anti-inflammatory and antioxidant benefits (Kumar et al., 2010).

Go for organic as non-organic cucumbers are commonly found with high levels of pesticide residue.

12. Sweet potato

These beautiful orange potatoes not only taste delicious but also are packed with carotenoids, which are being extensively researched for the role they play in fat development, obesity and weight-loss. This highly nutritious tuber is easily digestible and excellent to reduce inflammation of the digestive tract. Sweet potato also contains calcium, magnesium, potassium, folate, vitamin C and vitamin E. They are perfect to make into chips, use as a topping for cottage pie, grated into salads or added to curries.

13. Sweetcorn

Corn is an excellent food for the brain; it's a rich source of essential fats and magnesium, as well as iron, potassium, zinc and B3. If serving popped corn then add a mineral rich salt such as "Mineral Salt" (rich in organic micronutrient complexes) or Himalayan Rock Salt (rich in mineral complexes). Kids love listening to corn pop, so instead of buying the ready-made corn covered in additives and flavourings try making your own.

14. Buckwheat

Buckwheat is a gluten free grass; it is not classed as a cereal although it is used in cereals, pancakes, pasta, noodles and bread. Buckwheat contains eight amino acids making it an excellent vegetarian protein. It is high in phosphorus, beta-carotene, vitamin C, calcium, magnesium, potassium, zinc, manganese and folate, as well as the flavonoids rutin and quercitin (Natural Standards Database, 2014). It's perfect for gastric band wearers as it is easy to swallow and has quite a distinct flavour.

15. Coconut oil

Coconut oil has been eaten for its health and nutritional benefits around the world for centuries. Coconut oil contains medium chain fatty acids (MCFAs), which are rapidly used by the liver to make energy. Virgin coconut oil (the oil extracted from fresh coconut meat) contains more MCFAs than non-virgin oil and has been shown to reduce abdominal fat (Liau et al., 2011). The lauric acid in coconut oil is used by the body to make monolaurin, a disease-fighting fatty acid, which is antimicrobial and able to deactivate bacteria, yeast, fungi and viruses (Enig, 1996).

Coconut oil satisfies the appetite and can help balance blood sugar levels by slowing the release of glucose from food in to the bloodstream. This healthy fat has been shown to support heart health, it's great for cooking as it remains stable at higher temperatures (so better to use than vegetable oils which become damaged with heat), and can be used as a dairy-free alternative to butter.

Note: Coconut oil, coconut milk, and fresh and desiccated coconut all have the properties mentioned above.

16. Fennel

Fennel digests fats well and acts as an antispasmodic, relieves stomach cramps and stomach pains. Fennel is also used to alleviate constipation, excessive hair growth (hirsutism), and nausea (Natural Standards Database, 2014). Rich in folate, vitamin C, potassium and phytoestrogens.

17. Seaweed

Seaweeds, also known as algaes, are a wonderful marine medicinal food. They are an excellent source of vitamins including A, B, C and E; as well as minerals including calcium, iodine, iron and potassium. Seaweeds are commonly used for cleansing the body of toxins and aiding digestion. Seaweed is also a high fibre food, and this fibre helps you feel fuller faster and reduces the appetite, it acts as a prebiotic and reduces inflammation in the digestive tract (Rajapakse & Kim, 2011).

Current research is investigating the properties from red, brown and green seaweeds as many of them have been shown to have therapeutic properties for health management, including anti-obesity, anti-diabetic, anti-hypertensive, anti-hyperlipidaemia, antioxidant, anti-inflammatory, immune-modulatory, thyroid stimulating, antibacterial and tissue healing properties (Miyashita, 2009; Mohamed et al., 2012)

18. Melon

Melons should be eaten alone for maximum benefit. They are high in water and an excellent cleansing and rehydrating food. Perfect for gastric band wearers.

19. Quinoa

Gluten free. Commonly known as a grain but is actually a seed, quinoa is easy to digest and a good vegetarian protein. It contains lysine (a potent antiviral agent), calcium (more than milk), iron, magnesium, phosphorus and potassium as well as B3. It may be used instead of rice or pasta.

20. Protein powders (pea, whey, hemp, rice)

Protein satisfies hunger more than fat or carbohydrate, increases weight-loss, and helps prevent weight gain (Bendtsen et al., 2013). Protein induces satiety, increases gastrointestinal hormone secretion, and is thermogenic (increases energy expenditure by raising the metabolic rate).

Protein powders are a convenient and easy way for someone with a gastric band to increase their protein intake, bearing in mind the restricted capacity of the banded stomach. Protein powders can be mixed into a smoothie for breakfast; these smoothies are a really good way to start the day. Protein powder can also be added to soups, savoury muffins or as a substitute for breadcrumbs in homemade burgers.

5.7 *Hydration*

Fruits and vegetables contain large amounts of water and nutrients in proportion to their weight. These are foods we recommend to enhance your hydration and nutrient status. Add more of these foods to your diet if you are feeling dehydrated or constipated.

Name of vegetable or fruit and percentage of water content:

Vegetables

1. Cucumber	96%
2. Lettuce	96%
3. Celery	95%
4. Radish	95%
5. Courgette	95%
6. Tomato	94%
7. Cabbage green	93%
8. Cabbage red	92%
9. Sweet peppers	92%
10. Cauliflower	92%
11. Spinach	92%
12. Broccoli	91%
13. Carrot	87%
14. Fresh peas	79%

Fruit

1. Watermelon	92%
2. Strawberries	92%
3. Grapefruit	91%
4. Cantaloupe	90%
5. Peach	88%
6. Raspberry	87%

7. Pineapple	87%
8. Orange	87%
9. Cranberry	87%
10. Apricot	86%
11. Blueberry	85%
12. Plum	85%
13. Apple	84%
14. Grapes	81%

Source: Pennington & Spungen (2010) Bowes and Church's Food Values of Portions Commonly used. 19th Edn. Lippincott, Williams and Wilkins, Philadelphia.

Summary:

- ✓ What changes do you feel comfortable making with your food, drink and the quality of both?
- ✓ Think about why, what and how you are eating. What can you change?
- ✓ Become familiar with the three phases, move in and out of them at your own pace
- ✓ Eat three meals a day and don't graze
- ✓ Chew each mouthful really well – count the number of times to slow you down
- ✓ Focus on eating – sit and eat at a table, ban phones, TV's and computers from meal times, be aware of what you are eating and savour it
- ✓ Eat in a relaxed state
- ✓ Eat slowly – put your fork or spoon down between mouthfuls
- ✓ Use small plates and bowls
- ✓ Take small mouthfuls - use a teaspoon or child's fork
- ✓ Listen to your body – are you still hungry or have you had enough to eat?
- ✓ Why are you eating – are you hungry or are you upset, anxious, angry or happy?
- ✓ Watch out for sauces, drinking excess calories and sugar in ready-made foods
- ✓ Choose some of the foods you'd like to include from our Twenty Foods for Gastric Band Wearers list
- ✓ If you are feeling dehydrated come back to the Hydrating Foods list

Chapter 6

Nutrients

> *If we are creating ourselves all the time, then it is never too late to begin creating the bodies we want instead of the ones we mistakenly assume we are stuck with.*
>
> Deepak Chopra

The foods we get the majority of our energy from can be divided in to three primary groups: proteins, fats and carbohydrates.

6.1 Protein, fats, carbohydrates and water

Protein not only makes you feel fuller for longer but also is essential to build and repair the body, and is in the inner and outer membrane of every cell. Protein comes in many different forms and has multiple functions in the body including the production of your DNA, neurotransmitters, enzymes, blood, bone, muscle, and hair, skin and nails. Protein is found in meat, fish, nuts, seeds, beans and dairy.

Fats support a number of our body's functions including helping to maintain normal heart function, absorbing and transporting vitamins A, D, E and K through the bloodstream, providing energy, forming a structural component of the brain, protecting our organs and nerves, providing the essential fatty acids that cannot be made by the body, and forming steroid hormones that are required to regulate many processes in the body. Dietary fats are found in nuts, seeds, fish, eggs, plants, meat and dairy.

Carbohydrates are the body's preferred energy source and are used before protein, fat and alcohol. Complex carbohydrates (vegetables and whole grains) retain their nutrients as well as fibre; the fibre makes them harder to digest, slowing the release of energy into the bloodstream, as well as providing vital food for our beneficial gut bacteria. Refined carbohydrates such as white bread, rice and pasta are digested quickly which can lead to problems with blood sugar control and fatigue.

Water keeps the body's temperature normal, nourishes and protects the brain and other tissues, lubricates joints, moves nutrients around the body to where they are needed, and helps the removal of waste through perspiration, the bowel and urine. Too much water can be dangerous, as can too little. Our requirement for water depends on the climate we live in and how physically active we are. The best way to decide if you are getting enough is to check the colour of your urine – if it is very pale yellow you are probably drinking enough, if it is dark yellow you may need more.

Contrary to common beliefs, the obese individual is not well nourished. (Lo Menzo et al., 2014)

6.2 Vitamins and Minerals

Vitamins are needed for normal growth and function, and as the body cannot make vitamins we must get them from our food. Becoming deficient in any vitamin damages our health. Vitamins cannot be digested and metabolised without the aid of minerals and the body doesn't manufacture a single mineral.

A vitamin is a substance that makes you ill if you don't eat it.

Albert Szent-Gyorgyi, Nobel Prize in Physiology or Medicine, 1937

Minerals are needed for maintaining normal health and are all essential (we can't make them so have to eat foods that contain them, i.e. plants, animals and water). Minerals are required for strong bones and teeth, skin and hair, blood, nerve and muscle function, and metabolic processes such as digestion.

There is a high prevalence of nutrient deficiencies in candidates BEFORE they have bariatric surgery (Aasheim et al., 2008; Ernst et al., 2009; Schweiger et al., 2010; Lo Menzo et al., 2014), and research shows a real risk for nutritional deficiencies for the band wearer (Fish et al., 2010).

Micronutrients – Some Pre-op Data:

Flancbaum et al., (2006) measured pre operative nutrient status of a group of 379 patients (320 women and 59 men) with mean BMIs between 40-60kg/m² and found:

43.9% were iron deficient (more common in younger patients)
8.4% were ferritin deficient (more common in women)
22% were haemoglobin deficient (with nearly twice as many men being deficient as women)
29% were thiamine deficient
68.1% were vitamin D deficient

Gimmel et al., (2009) studied 312 patients with an average BMI of 52.3 kg/m² and found that:

57.4% were vitamin D deficient (more common in Hispanics and blacks)
12.5% were vitamin A deficient
3.5% were B12 deficient
23.5% fit the criteria of hyperparathyroidism

Routine screening of obese people before bariatric surgery has shown multiple micronutrient deficiencies so here is an overview of nutrients and why you need them in your life. This section has been written out alphabetically, not in the order of importance.

There is a high prevalence of nutrient deficiencies in candidates BEFORE they have bariatric surgery.

6.3 Why we need it, signs of deficiency, and foods to include

6.3.1 Calcium

Gastric band wearers are recommended to supplement with additional calcium citrate – see chapter 8 for more details. Calcium deficiency occurs because the stomach pouch produces little or no acid necessary for optimal calcium absorption. It is advisable to have your bone density or bone mineral turnover measured at frequent intervals. The frequency will depend on your initial results.

> **It is advisable to have your bone density or bone turnover measured at frequent intervals.**

The body needs calcium to maintain strong bones, for muscle movement, and for nerves to carry messages between the brain and every part of the body. Calcium helps blood vessels move blood throughout the body and helps release hormones and enzymes that affect almost every function of the body. Almost all calcium is stored in bones and teeth, where it supports their structure and hardness (Office of Dietary Supplements, 2013).

Signs of calcium deficiency include:

- Bone loss – osteoporosis, osteomalacia, rickets
- Hypertension and irregularities in muscle, heart, or nerve functions
- Tingling fingers

- Defects in certain hormones
- Weight gain

Foods to include:

Milk, yogurt and cheese contain high amounts of calcium but, for the lactose or dairy intolerant person, tinned fish with soft bones (such as salmon or sardines), tofu, shrimp and green leafy veg such as kale, broccoli and Chinese cabbage are also good sources.

But be cautious of: Caffeine, carbonated drinks, and alcohol as they effect calcium excretion.

A number of medications interact with calcium levels in the body, including antibiotics, oral contraceptives, antacids, diuretics, laxatives and glucocorticoids (Office of Dietary Supplements, 2013). It is essential that you are aware of any interactions and that you share your full medical history with your health practitioner.

6.3.2 Chromium

Chromium deficiency is common in bariatric surgery candidates, and concentrations are lower in those with a higher BMI (Lima et al., 2013). Chromium supplementation helps reduce weight, binge eating and symptoms of depression (Brownley et al., 2013), along with increasing insulin sensitivity and lowering blood glucose in those with type 2 diabetes (Brownley et al., 2015).

Chromium activates enzymes involved in glucose (blood sugar) metabolism and stabilises blood sugar levels, cleans the arteries by reducing cholesterol and triglyceride levels, helps transport amino acids to where the body needs them, and helps control the appetite. Medical research has shown that people with low levels of chromium in their bodies are more susceptible to cancer, heart problems, and diabetes. Deficiency may result in glucose intolerance in diabetics, arteriosclerosis, heart disease, obesity, and tiredness.

Signs of Chromium Deficiency:

- Food cravings

- Diabetes

- High cholesterol

- Hypoglycaemia

- Glucose intolerance

Foods to include:

Meat (particularly liver), cheese, and whole grains.

6.3.3 Copper

Copper deficiency is more common in women and even more so in women in their 50s and 60s. Risk factors for becoming deficient in copper include bariatric surgery (although mostly found in RYGB), overloading in zinc and iron supplements, and coeliac disease (Jaiser & Winston, 2010).

Copper is necessary for the body to absorb and use iron to make red blood cells, is important in maintaining myelin (a fatty substance covering some nerves) and is needed for taste sensitivity. Copper is also a component of connective tissue, cartilage and skin, and helps proper bone formation, development and maintenance. Copper is also required for energy production and the immune system.

If you have raised homocysteine it may be worth getting your copper levels checked too (Jaiser & Winston, 2010).

Signs of copper deficiency may include:

- Anaemia

- Depression

- Poor immunity

- Worsening eye sight

- Peripheral neuropathy (ends of fingers and toes feeling numb or lack of feeling)

- Bone defects or gait difficulties

- Cognitive dysfunction

Foods to include:

Liver, shellfish, meat, nuts, legumes, whole grains, and raisins.

6.3.4 Iodine

Being obese is an independent risk factor for iodine deficiency (Lecube et al., 2015).

Iodine, an essential trace element, is vital for healthy thyroid function. The thyroid gland regulates the body's production of energy, physical and mental growth, nervous system function, circulation and metabolism of all nutrients.

To make thyroid hormones it is essential that the thyroid gland has the right amount of iodine. Iodine deficiency is one of the three most common micronutrient deficiencies in the world today (World Health Organisation). Our bodies don't make iodine, we have to get it from our food. Having too much iodine, as well as too little, can cause or worsen hypothyroidism. A simple urine test can measure your iodine level.

Signs of an iodine deficiency may include:

- Goiter
- Hypothyroidism – low thyroid function (see chapter 3 for detailed information)
- Mental impairment

Foods to include:

Seaweed (whole or sheet), watercress, haddock, shrimp and lobster, cod, low fat plain yogurt, iodized salt, semi-skimmed milk, egg, lean braising steak.

Iodine Deficiency

In 2004, it was estimated that of the 2 billion people around the world at risk of iodine deficiency, 20% live in Europe. Of considerable concern are the subtle degrees of mental impairment associated with iodine deficiency that lead to poor school performance, reduced intellectual ability, and impaired work capacity (WHO, 2007).

6.3.5 Iron

Patients scheduled for bariatric surgery have an estimated 10-15% prevalence of anaemia, 30-40% prevalence of iron deficiency (may or may not also be anaemic) (Ignacio, 2013) and 18 months post-gastric band surgery 72% of patients were iron deficient (Harris & Barger, 2010).

Iron is needed for all body functions, which is why every cell in our bodies contains and needs it. The majority of our iron is in our red blood cells in the form of haemoglobin, which carries oxygen from our lungs to the rest of our body. A small amount of iron is found in our muscles in the form of myoglobin, which carries and stores our muscles' oxygen.

Iron is critical for energy production so it's not surprising that iron deficiency and iron deficiency anaemia are associated with decreased physical endurance and exercise capacity (Crouter et al., 2013). A poor ability to exercise may be due to iron deficiency.

Poor nutrition is one of the main reasons for iron deficiency, along with repeated dieting (Pinhas-Hamiel et al., 2003). Interestingly, the prevalence of iron deficiency increases with body mass index and iron absorption is affected by an increased BMI and inflammation (Eftekhari et al., 2009; McClung & Karl, 2009). So simply put, being overweight or obese increases your risk of being iron deficient, and being iron deficient increases your risk of being overweight or obese.

Obese people often have iron-deficiency anaemia pre-operatively (Fish et al., 2010) and the band makes it even harder to meet nutritional needs post-op. There is a reported 30%-57% prevalence of anaemia in patients having had restrictive-type surgery and iron deficiency in 72% of patients 18 months after band placement (Harris & Barger, 2010). Iron deficiencies occur after adjustable gastric banding because of decreased intake of iron rich foods, particularly in the early postoperative stages, or due to poor compliance with supplementation. Therefore, iron status should be monitored. Excess amounts of iron can result in toxicity and even death (Office of Dietary Supplements, 2013). It is recommended that appropriate medical and nutritional evaluation should be sought prior to iron supplementation (Linus Pauling Institute, 2013).

Being overweight or obese increases your risk of being iron deficient, and being iron deficient increases your risk of being overweight or obese.

Anaemia is either a reduction in the number of red blood cells being produced, or of haemoglobin in the blood. This results in reduced levels of oxygen being transported round the body, which is vital for every cell to produce energy for movement.

Anaemia can stem from a deficiency in iron, which can result from poor absorption or low dietary intake, increased iron requirement (for example during growth or menstruation), and excessive blood loss (possibly due to injury or surgery). Vitamin B12 is also needed to prevent anaemia, which works with folate in regulating the formation of red blood cells, and helps to utilise iron.

> **It may be advisable to get a Full Blood Count via your GP or a specific test for Anaemia via a Registered Nutritional Therapist.**

Signs of Iron Deficiency may include:

- Fatigue
- Irritability
- Paleness
- Difficulty swallowing
- Heart palpitations during exertion
- Lack of well-being
- Craving for salt
- Poor learning ability
- Poor endurance
- Low tolerance for cold
- Faulty attention span
- Frequent infections
- Reduced white blood cell counts
- Impaired antibody production

Foods to include:

Heme Iron - Meat sources:

Liver, meat, turkey, chicken, fish, crab (Alaskan fresh)

Non-heme Iron - Plant sources:

Eggs, leafy veg (i.e. spinach, cabbage), sesame seeds, soybeans, lentils, kidney beans, almonds, prunes, hummus, peas, and molasses.

> **Vitamin C strongly enhances the absorption of non–heme (plant sources) iron.**

But be cautious of:

Phytates found in beans, lentils and grains as these inhibit absorption, as does soya protein, tea, coffee and wine (Linus Pauling Institute, 2013). However, soaking pulses and grains overnight before cooking will help to break down the phytic acid, and is recommended.

What else should I know?

Vitamin A deficiency makes iron deficiency anaemia worse.

Copper is needed for iron metabolism, so sometimes anaemia is a clinical sign of copper deficiency.

Calcium can decrease the absorption of iron so supplements should not be taken together (Linus Pauling Institute, 2013).

A number of medications may impair iron absorption, including antacids and proton pump inhibitors. It is essential that you are aware of any interactions and that you share your full medical history with your health practitioner.

6.3.6 Manganese

Manganese is important in the blood breakdown of amino acids and the production of energy, and activates enzymes, which are important for proper digestion and utilisation of foods. Manganese plays a role in blood sugar control, which is important for weight management.

Manganese is also a catalyst in the breakdown of fats and cholesterol, helps nourish the nerves and brain, and maintains sex hormone production, bone development and collagen formation (Missouri Bariatric Service, 2011; Shultz et al., 2004).

Signs of Manganese deficiency include:

- Loss of hearing
- Skin rashes
- Digestive problems
- Decreased hair and nail growth
- Poor carbohydrate and fat metabolism
- Loss of hair colour

Foods to include:

Pecans, brazil nuts, almond, buckwheat, split peas, fresh spinach, oats, rhubarb, Brussels sprouts, carrot, broccoli, seeds, avocados, seaweed, whole grains. Cloves, ginger, thyme, and bay leaves are also high in manganese so it is worth adding these spices and herbs to your cooking.

6.3.7 Magnesium

Higher levels of magnesium intake are correlated with reduced abdominal obesity, protection against metabolic syndrome, and improvements in glucose control for those with type 2 diabetes (Watson & Preedy, 2012).

Magnesium is critical for proper cell function and activates at least 300 hundred enzymes throughout the body. Along with calcium, vitamin D and vitamin K2, magnesium is needed for strong, healthy bones and teeth so is important for band wearers due to risk of osteoporosis. Magnesium is also involved in energy regulation and metabolism, helps muscles relax, is anti-inflammatory, affects muscle tone of blood vessels, is important in maintaining nerve function and is involved in proper insulin production.

Conditions that may involve magnesium deficiency include:

- Angina
- Asthma
- Cardiovascular disease
- Irregular heartbeat
- Diabetes
- Insulin resistance
- Fatigue
- Kidney Stones
- Migraines
- PMS
- Fibromyalgia
- Osteoporosis
- High blood pressure

Foods to include:

Kelp, whole grains, almonds, cashew nuts, blackstrap molasses, dulse, meat, seafood, millet, pecan nuts, beans, dandelion greens, garlic, fresh green peas, banana, sweet potato, and blackberries.

Note: If you frequently use antacids or laxatives then you may have insufficient magnesium levels (Shulz et al., 2004).

6.3.8 Potassium

Potassium is the most abundant electrolyte found in the body. It works with sodium to regulate the body's waste balance and normalise heart rhythms as well as maintaining fluid balance in our cells. It is used to convert glucose (blood sugar) into glycogen for storage, assists in reducing high blood pressure, and also aids nerve transmission, muscle contraction and hormone secretion. When dehydrated more potassium is lost through the urine and should be a consideration for gastric band wearers who can be constantly thirsty and feel dehydrated.

Signs of Potassium Deficiency:

- High blood pressure
- Nausea
- Vomiting
- Muscle weakness or spasms
- Tachycardia (rapid heartbeat)

Foods to include:

Seaweeds such as dulse and kelp, sunflower seeds, almonds, parsley, brazil nuts, dates, figs, avocado, pecan, yam, Swiss chard, cooked soy bean, garlic, spinach, walnuts, millet, beans, mushrooms, winter squash, celery, and radish.

Note: Potassium intake may need to be restricted in people taking potassium-sparing diuretics or ACE inhibitors (Shultz et al., 2004).

6.3.9 Selenium

Selenium levels have been shown to be reduced after having gastric band surgery, therefore supplementation with selenium is recommended for at least the first three months after surgery (Freeth et al., 2012).

Selenium is an essential mineral and major antioxidant that protects cell membranes and prevents free radical generation leading to a decreased risk of degenerative diseases such as heart disease. Studies also show that selenium is helpful in reducing symptoms related to arthritis by helping reduce swelling in joints. Selenium also preserves tissue elasticity, slows down the ageing and hardening of tissues and improves skin conditions such as acne and dandruff. Selenium has been shown to be protective against environmental toxicity from chemicals and heavy metals such as mercury and arsenic.

Signs of Selenium deficiency are similar to those of vitamin E and may include:

- Muscular weakness
- Reduced immune function
- Premature aging
- Rheumatoid arthritis
- Heart disease

Foods to include:

Seafood, meat, whole grains, Brazil nuts, apple cider vinegar, scallops, lobster, red Swiss chard, oats, clams, king crab, cod, brown rice, black strap molasses, garlic.

The amount of selenium in foods depends on the animals' diet and the selenium content of the soil the foods are grown in (Shultz et al., 2004).

6.3.10 Vitamin A

Obese individuals have been found to have a lower intake as well as lower vitamin A levels compared to healthy weight people (Garcia, 2012).

Vitamin A is a fat-soluble vitamin involved in vision, bone growth, reproduction and cell division, it is also important for the immune system and is required for detoxification of environmental pollutants. Vitamin A requires fat as well as other minerals to be properly absorbed by your digestive system.

> *Vitamin A deficiency increases the risk of fat deposition and inflammation.*
>
> Garcia, 2012

Signs of Vitamin A deficiency may include:

- Night blindness or deteriorating eyesight
- Poor skin tone or maybe acne, boils, superficial wrinkles or age spots
- Lowered immune function
- Respiratory infections

Vitamin A comes in two forms either as retinol from animal products and as carotene (known as pro-vitamin A as it needs to be converted in the body to vitamin A).

Foods to include:

Vitamin A – Animal Sources

Liver, non-fat fortified milk, cheddar cheese, and eggs.

Vitamin A – Plant Sources (beta carotene)

Dark green and brightly coloured veg such as sweet potato baked in skin, carrot, spinach, kale, melon, and romaine lettuce.

Note: Vitamin A from animal foods are better absorbed than from plants.

6.3.11 Vitamin B1 (Thiamine)

Vitamin B1 deficiency is common after all types of bariatric surgery, including the gastric band, but especially after rapid weight-loss. If you persistently vomit, which is a common side effect (Chavallier, 2010), thiamine must be supplemented (Dixon, 2001).

At least two cases have been reported of severe B1 deficiency (Wernicke's Encephalopathy) post gastric banding and the risks appear to be highest within the first 4-12 weeks post-surgery, and in particular in young women with frequent vomiting (Singh & Kumar, 2007).

Deficiencies may also occur if meals are skipped or if the appropriate vitamins are not taken. Thiamine stores in the body are very small and daily replenishment is required.

Deficiencies in thiamine can have some very serious consequences as thiamine deficiency significantly affects the central nervous system.

Signs of Vitamin B1 Deficiency:

* Fatigue
* Apathy
* Poor concentration

- Poor memory
- Insomnia
- Loss of appetite
- Emotional instability
- Irritability
- Racing heart
- Depression
- Poor detoxification

Foods to include:

Sunflower seeds, liver, pine nuts, pork, dried beans, peas, beans, whole grains, egg yolk, turkey, chicken, and fish.

Note: Diets high in sugar and fat usually lead to a low thiamine intake (Shultz et al., 2004).

6.3.12 Vitamin B6 (Pyridoxine)

Obese people have significantly lower levels of vitamin B6 than healthy weight people (Aasheim et al., 2008). B6 is involved in the metabolism of amino acids and essential fatty acids so is needed for growth and maintenance of nearly all the structures and functions in the body. B6 is especially important for a healthy nervous system, red blood cell metabolism, cardiovascular health, immune health and women's health.

Note: Taking an oral contraceptive can lower levels of B6.

Signs of a B6 deficiency may include:

- Depression and emotional illness
- Anaemia

- High homocysteine
- Heart attack
- PMS
- Fertility problems
- Acne
- Dermatitis

Foods to include:

Sunflower seeds, pistachio nuts, fish, turkey and chicken, prunes, eggs, avocado, spinach, bananas, wheat germ.

6.3.13 Vitamin B12 (Cobalamin)

Vitamin B12 deficiency is associated with being overweight or obese (Baltaci et al., 2013).

Vitamin B12 is needed to form healthy blood and is involved in producing myelin (a fatty substance in a sheath covering our nerves).

Deficiency in vitamin B12, if left untreated, can cause a number of health problems such as loss of mental alertness, neuropathies, nausea, muscle weakness, digestive upset, depression, irritability, memory impairment, poor concentration and water retention.

Because certain medications, such as metformin and proton pump inhibitors (PPIs), can decrease the availability of vitamin B12 for absorption, additional supplementation may be required after surgery. Only 1% of vitamin B12 taken orally is absorbed. Vitamin B12 is best absorbed when taken sublingually (dissolved completely under the tongue) or as an injection.

Signs of Vitamin B12 Deficiency:

- Pallor
- Fatigue
- High homocysteine
- Confusion
- Memory loss
- Depression

Note: If you have been under considerable stress your need for B12 and other B vitamins may be increased.

Foods to include:

Kidney, liver, beef, mackerel, sardines, herring, egg yolk, trout, brains, salmon, tuna, lamb, whey protein, Edam, Swiss, Brie, and Blue cheese.

6.3.14 Vitamin B9 (Folate)

One study found that 2 years post gastric banding, patients' folate levels had declined by 44% (Gasteyger et al., 2006).

Folate is profoundly far-reaching in the body; it participates in the production of neurotransmitters, the production of DNA and RNA, the immune system, and the formation of red blood cells.

Folic acid is the synthetic form of folate and must be transformed in the body to methyl-folate before it is active and can be used. Folic acid that has not been converted will build up in the system and block folate transportation around the body and block folate receptors. The inactive folic acid will deny access to the cell of the active folate so the cells will pull folic acid in instead, resulting in a folate deficiency (Lynch, 2014).

Malabsorption and certain medications, such as anticonvulsants, oral contraceptives and cancer treating agents, can also be responsible for folate deficiency. Low prenatal levels in mothers can cause neural tube defects in newborns.

Folate, Folic Acid, Folinic acid and L-methyl folate - simplified.

- Folate is a natural vitamin found in foods, mainly green leafy vegetables i.e. foliage! It is also made in the human digestive tract.
- Folic acid is a synthetic form of folate that is widely used as a supplement. This causes problems in people with a defect MTHFR gene (approximately 40-60% of the population).
- Folinic acid is an intermediately form between folic acid and the most bioavailable form L-Methyl folate.
- L-methyl folate is the most bioavailable form on the market. (Wilson, 2014)

Note: If supplementing folate, make sure it is in the form of L-Methylfolate. The supplement name you are looking for is L 5 methyl-tetrahydrofolate or 5 formyl tetrahydrofolate. Due to various interactions it is still advisable to take a B-complex rather than supplementing single vitamins unless you are working with a nutritional professional.

Signs of folate deficiency:

- Anxiety
- Depression
- High homocysteine
- Frequent illness
- Folic acid anaemia (characterised by oversized red blood cells)

Foods to include:

Black eyed peas, lentils, dark green leafy veg (spinach, kale, savoy cabbage), asparagus, lettuce, avocado, fresh coconut, mushrooms, and blackberries.

6.3.15 Vitamin C

Obese people have significantly lower levels of vitamin C than healthy weight people (Aasheim et al., 2008) and depletion or deficiency is common in people prior to bariatric surgery (Reiss et al., 2009).

There is conflicting data over vitamin C deficiencies seen in patients after having a gastric band fitted, with one study finding no decrease in vitamin C levels (Aasheim et al., 2008) and another finding that 35% of patients were deficient, and that was at one year and two years postoperatively (Clements et al., 2006).

Deficiencies in vitamin C lead to symptoms that include:

- Bleeding gums
- Weakness
- Lowered immunity

- Irritability
- Muscle and joint pains
- Poor dental health

Foods to include:

Broccoli, Brussel sprouts, black currants, kale, sweet peppers, cabbage, and cauliflower.

6.3.16 Vitamin D

Between 25 – 80% of adult pre-bariatric patients may have baseline vitamin D deficiency (Xanthakos, 2009)

Barely a day passes when we don't hear someone talking about vitamin D and it seems to be hailed as the new wonder vitamin. We are not going so far as to say that, but clinical research has confirmed that there is a worldwide problem with vitamin D depletion.

Vitamin D is a fat-soluble vitamin and can be made when your skin is exposed to sunlight; it is needed by nearly every cell of the body and helps calcium absorption in the intestine. Low fat diets and sedentary lifestyles may contribute to a lower intake (Adams & Hewison, 2010; Brock et al., 2010).

A recent nationwide survey in the UK showed that more than 50% of the adult population has insufficient levels and that 16% have severe deficiency during winter and spring (Pearce & Cheetham, 2010).

The National Health and Nutrition Examination Survey showed that the only trend that matched vitamin D depletion was an increase in obesity (Yetley, 2008). Hewison (Adams & Hewison, 2010) has unpublished data, which shows that when mice are vitamin D deficient they have an increase in body weight, and in 2009, Foss proposed in Medical Hypotheses that vitamin D deficiency is the cause of common obesity.

Vitamin D is stored in body fat compartments, however it is not as available for the body to use when you are obese, as it has been "trapped" in the fat cells. When levels rise vitamin D slowly becomes more available to the body (Adams & Hewison, 2010; Brock et al., 2010; Wortman et al., 2003).

Safe sun light exposure is the primary source of vitamin D but it is also found in small amounts in oily fish such as salmon, mackerel, herring (with wild salmon having 4-5 times as much vitamin D in it than farmed salmon) and the oils from fish such as cod liver oil (Holick & Chen, 2008). Foods are also fortified with vitamin D, however you may like to check if this is the most bioavailable form (D3) or the cheaper form (D2) added. Vitamin D2 is only 30-50% as effective as D3. Vigorous physical exercise has also been shown to contribute to vitamin D levels (Brock et al., 2010).

Supplements are available but check the label to ensure it is D3 prior to purchase. We recommend testing your level prior to supplementation, restoring vitamin D status as the first priority, then maintaining this level. The best method for testing is to measure 25(OH)D concentrations. Tests are available via your GP or Registered Nutritional Therapist.

Signs of vitamin D deficiency may include:

- Rickets – associated symptoms of stunted growth and bone deformity
- Osteomalacia – weakened muscles and bones
- Weak immune system
- Poor hair growth

Best source of vitamin D is SUNSHINE!

Amount depends on many factors including location, season and skin colour but about 10,000IU can be made in the skin upon around 15 minutes of sun exposure.

Foods to include:

Oily fish (sea bass, salmon, halibut, herring, trout), mushrooms, caviar, egg yolk.

6.3.17 Vitamin E

Obese people have significantly lower levels of Vitamin E than healthy weight people (Aasheim et al., 2008).

Vitamin E is a fat-soluble antioxidant, which plays a diverse role in our health, including immune function, cell-signalling, and gene expression (Traver et al., 2006). Importantly for band wearers, vitamin E has been shown to reduce inflammation, improve liver function and improve insulin function. Other potential benefits include preventing many age-related diseases such as cardiovascular disease, reducing cholesterol and alleviating symptoms of PMS (Manning et al., 2004; Jiang, 2014; Natural Standards Database, 2014).

Signs of Vitamin E deficiency may include:

- Lethargy
- Poor concentration
- Poor wound healing
- Susceptibility to infections
- Apathy
- Irritability
- Muscle weakness

Foods to include:

Vitamin E occurs in the fats of vegetable foods with natural (unprocessed) vegetable oils being the richest sources: wheat germ oil, sunflower seeds, almonds and hazelnuts. If using vegetable oils for your vitamin E, choose cold-pressed or unrefined. Vitamin E is also found in whole grains, spinach, broccoli, mango, kiwi, and tomatoes (Office of Dietary Supplements, 2014).

Vitamin E in Spinach

½ cup cooked spinach = 1.9mg

1 cup raw spinach = 0.6mg

6.3.18 Vitamin K

In 2008 a case was reported where a woman, pregnant 2 years after gastric banding, had prolonged vomiting due to her band slipping, this resulted in *"extensive intracranial foetal hemorrhage due to maternal vitamin K deficiency"*. The authors of this case stressed the importance of vitamin substitution (Van Mieghem et al., 2008).

Vitamin K is a fat-soluble vitamin and comes in three forms, K1 (found in plants), K2 (made by gut bacteria and found in animal foods) and K3 (a synthetic form). Vitamin K1 is required for healthy blood clotting. Vitamin K2 is particularly important for band wearers due to its critical role in building strong bones as it helps move calcium from the blood into bones and teeth. Vitamin K is often included in very small doses or not at all in multivitamins due to the fact that it may interfere with anticoagulation medications, such as Warfarin. Gut bacteria make around 50% of our vitamin K so a healthy gut is important (Shultz et al., 2004).

Discuss with your health practitioner an appropriate level of dietary vitamin K if you take anticoagulants.

Signs of a vitamin K deficiency may include:

- Bleeding and clotting disorders
- Calcification of the blood vessels

Foods to include:

Vitamin K1: carrots, celery, berries, green leafy veg (kale, spinach, broccoli, cabbage), tomatoes.

Vitamin K2: grass-fed organic animal products (i.e. eggs, butter, Brie and Gouda cheese, chicken drumsticks), some fermented foods (such as natto) and goose liver pate.

6.3.19 Zinc

Zinc deficiency has been reported at around 28% prior to bariatric surgery (Xanthakos, 2009).

Zinc is an antioxidant nutrient necessary for protein synthesis, wound healing, prostate functions, and male hormone activity. Also, zinc regulates muscle contractility, is important for blood stability, maintains the body's alkaline balance, helps in normal tissue function, and aids in the digestion and metabolism of phosphorus.

Symptoms of deficiency may include:

- Prolonged healing of wounds
- White spots on fingernails
- Stretch marks
- Fatigue
- Decreased alertness
- Susceptibility to infections

Foods to include:

Meat, fish, seafood, liver, eggs, legumes, and whole grains.

Summary:

✓ Read through the vitamins and minerals noting any deficiencies you think you may have.

✓ If you think you may have a number of nutrient deficiencies consider having a nutritional evaluation test.

✓ Which foods are you comfortable to try, add or increase into your daily life?

✓ If your symptoms persist or are severe please seek support from your bariatric team or health care provider.

Chapter 7

Supplements

Gastric band wearers require supplements and therefore this chapter is a short summary of the most up-to-date evidence for the 'average' gastric band wearer. However, supplement plans should ideally be tailored around your specific health requirements and needs. We recommend speaking to your bariatric team or Registered Nutritional Therapist before making changes to your supplement programme.

> *Although there is a growing body of research in the field of weight-loss surgery most current recommendations for the care of weight-loss patients is based on case reports, non-randomized, small sample, retrospective studies and expert opinion. To date there is no standardisation of care between centres.*
>
> Mitchell & de Zwaan, 2011

Whilst the weight-loss associated with gastric bands is generally successful, there are some health implications, namely nutrient deficiencies that can lead to illness or disease (Fish et al., 2010). Obese patients often have vitamin D deficiency (Fish et al., 2010) and iron-deficiency anaemia pre-operatively and the band makes it even harder to meet nutritional needs post-op. Furthermore, changes in eating habits can result in low nutrient intake, therefore post-op supplementation should include vitamins, minerals and possibly protein (Buchwald, 2005).

> *A human being is a single being, unique and unrepeatable.*
>
> John Paul II

As discussed in chapter 6, routine screening of obese people before bariatric surgery has shown multiple deficiencies in micronutrients. The British Obesity & Metabolic Surgery Society (BOMSS) published new guidelines in September 2014 (O'Kane et al., 2014), recommending gastric band patients have the following blood tests **before surgery**:

- Full blood count
- Ferritin
- Folate
- Vitamin B12
- Vitamin D (25 hydroxy-vitamin D)
- Calcium
- Parathyroid hormone
- Liver function test
- Urea and electrolytes

Co-morbidities
- Fasting glucose
- HbA1c
- Lipid profile

Assuming that patients have received the above tests

preoperatively and that any nutritional deficiencies have been identified and treated, we recommend a minimum supplement programme as follows:

7.1 Minimum Supplement Programme:

✓ A good quality multivitamin supplement should include a range of vitamins including thiamine (vitamin B1), riboflavin (vitamin B2), nicotinic acid (vitamin B3), pantothenic acid (vitamin B5), pyridoxine (vitamin B6), biotin, folate (methylfolate or folinic acid), vitamin B12 and Vitamin E.

✓ Mineral supplement should include Iron, Zinc, Selenium, Copper, Manganese and Iodine

✓ Calcium citrate: 1,200 – 1,500 mg/day in divided doses

✓ Vitamin D3: as required after testing

✓ Folic acid*: 400ug/day minimum

✓ Vitamin B12 as needed

✓ Thiamine 200-300 mg daily (along with a strong vitamin B complex) *if patient experiences prolonged vomiting* – urgent referral to bariatric centre

✓ Selenium (for at least first 3 months post surgery)

(Dixon et al., 2001; Von Mach et al., 2004; O'Kane et al., 2014; Mechanick et al., 2013)

* Folic Acid – folic acid is a synthetic form of folate, it used to be the best we had but now there are vastly superior folate supplements in the form of methylfolate or folinic acid. These active forms of folate do not need to be transformed in the body like inactive folic acid, but can be used in their current form (Lynch, 2014).

Depending on how tight the band is and to prevent possible obstruction of the band, supplements may need to be in liquid, powder or chewable forms.

A number of studies have shown patients post-surgery have nutrient deficiencies yet there are also patients who have excess nutrient levels in their bodies. Supplementing in excess commonly causes this which is why we recommend to test, not guess.

7.1.1 Calcium

According to Von Mach et al., (2004), adjustable gastric band patients should take 1,200-1,500mg of calcium citrate daily in divided doses. In the light of recent research on calcium supplementation and possible increased risk of myocardial infarction (heart attack) (Li et al., 2012), it may be safer to focus on ensuring sufficient calcium is consumed through the diet to reduce an over reliance on calcium supplementation. Speak to your health professional for more personalised advice.

However, if you do take calcium supplements, the most effective form is calcium citrate, NOT calcium carbonate, phosphate, or coral calcium.

For optimal absorption, the calcium citrate should be taken with vitamin D3 (1,000-2,000 IU/day) (Kulick et al., 2010), ascorbic acid (vitamin C), magnesium and vitamin K2.

7.1.2 Magnesium

Adjustable gastric band patients should take a multivitamin with magnesium. Taking up to 300mg of magnesium per day may be necessary to correct deficiency (Massouri Bariatric Surgery, 2011).

7.1.3 Chromium

Having a band fitted does not stop the food cravings that may have contributed to the original weight gain. Therefore, it may be beneficial to have additional chromium supplementation. Chromium works with insulin in the metabolism of sugar and stabilises blood sugar levels, cleans the arteries by reducing cholesterol and triglyceride levels, helps transport amino acids to where the body needs them, and helps control the appetite.

7.1.4 Protein

Protein malnutrition is common in those who have had bariatric surgery (Coupaye et al., 2009), and protein may need to be supplemented in either liquid or powder form if you are unable to eat sufficient dietary protein.

We frequently recommend protein powder to our clients because they are a convenient and easily digestible source of protein. There are many different types of protein powder but we recommend pea, rice, hemp and whey protein. Protein powder can be mixed in to smoothies for breakfast, along with any other powder or liquid supplements.

7.1.5 Fibre

Fibre may be a consideration but caution is advised due to possible issues with sufficient water intake. If constipation is a problem, a fibre supplement such as psyllium or apple pectin might be helpful, or alternatively you can add a couple of tablespoons of chia or flaxseeds to your daily diet. Either way you must ensure you are drinking enough water or the additional fibre may make your constipation worse.

7.1.6 Anti-inflammatory Supplements

Overweight people have inflammation. Inflammation is a part of the body's immune response but systemic inflammation, especially over a long period of time, underlies many common diseases. Essential fatty acids are anti-inflammatory, particularly omega-3 essential fatty acids EPA and DHA, commonly found in fish oils.

Curcumin, the active compound in turmeric, is also anti-inflammatory.

7.1.7 Liver Support

The body stores toxins in fat tissue. As weight is lost, it may be beneficial to support the liver so it can cope with the extra burden of toxins being released. For more information on detoxification please refer to Chapter 3. If you would like a more personalised approach, please refer to your health professional.

7.1.8 Probiotics & Prebiotics

Please see chapter 3 for more detailed information on the role probiotics play in weight gain and loss.

If you are obese, have a history of antibiotic use, suffer with digestive issues or frequent illness, it may be beneficial to take a good quality multi-strain probiotic supplement. Probiotics are also found in some foods such as unpasteurised sauerkraut, kimchi, miso soup, 'live' yogurt and kefir.

Prebiotics are certain fibrous carbohydrates that feed the good bacteria in your gut and help it grow. Ideally eat them with probiotic rich foods or supplements. Focus on chicory, onions, leeks, garlic, oats, beans, lentils, chickpeas, bananas, asparagus and sweet potato.

NB: If you experience a reaction to eating these probiotic or prebiotic foods, our advice would be to stop eating them and only reintroduce them very slowly until your body acclimatises.

Summary:

✓ Ensure you receive full blood tests prior to surgery.

✓ Ensure you follow the recommended minimum supplement programme.

✓ Consider additional supplements where necessary.

✓ Speak to a health professional for personalised advice.

✓ Use the checklists in chapter 9 to keep track of your test results, medications if using and supplements.

Chapter 8

Recipes

In the kitchen

There are a few pieces of kitchen equipment we think are essential – a juicer, a blender and a slow cooker. See the checklist in Chapter 9 for more kitchen ideas.

The recipes here have been adapted to meet our nutritional recommendations but would comply with a little jiggling depending on what's in your fridge, so feel free to adapt them to your taste.

The size of the average stomach is 2 litres – that's pre-surgery. Post surgery your stomach will be between the size of a golf ball and a tennis ball. You will be the expert on your new stomach so listen to your body and stop eating when you feel full so you don't stretch your pouch. The amounts given in these recipes are approximate. We chose not to be prescriptive – we don't know if yours is a golf ball stomach or a tennis ball. Fresh ingredients vary hugely in size – there isn't an average sized carrot – so adapt the recipes to suit your stomach. Any leftovers can be kept in the fridge or freezer.

After surgery your stomach will be between the size of a golf ball and a tennis ball. Stop eating when you begin to feel full so you don't stretch your pouch.

8.1 Juices

Fresh juices are a great way of getting lots of nutrients in to your body with very little effort. Try different combinations to see which you like best but please don't overdo the fruit – add just enough to make the juice palatable – and focus on different coloured vegetables each day. Ideally a fresh juice would be drunk immediately but any leftover juice can be covered and kept in the fridge until the next day.

We recommend limited fruit in juices and smoothies to minimise the amount of glucose (sugar) entering your bloodstream. The body produces the hormone insulin in response to raised blood glucose. Over time, if the body is repeatedly exposed to too much sugar from foods (which can include fruit, all carbohydrate-rich foods such as bread, pasta and white rice as well as actual sugar), you can become resistant to insulin – this insulin resistance is the precursor to type 2 diabetes.

Berry Breakfast

1 large handful spinach
2 handfuls berries – strawberries, blueberries or raspberries
1 apple

'The Best' Green Juice

2 apples
½ cucumber
½ lemon, peeled
½ cup kale
½ cup spinach or kale
¼ bunch celery
1 inch piece of fresh ginger
¼ head of romaine lettuce

Cleansing Juice

3 large carrots
3 apples
1cm piece fresh ginger
1 beetroot

Fat Busting Juice

3 large grapefruit, peeled
1 cucumber
1 handful mint leaves

Alkalising Juice

1 cucumber
1 handful spinach or kale
Large bunch parsley
1 apple
1 stalk celery

Zingy Carrot Crush

6 carrots
1 inch piece of ginger
1 apple
1 lemon, peeled

Beet It

1 small beetroot
1 celery stalk
3 carrots
2 apples

Pineapple Passion

1 handful spinach or kale
1 handful fresh pineapple
1 handful parsley

8.2 Smoothies

There's no limit to the variations on smoothies so try experimenting with any of these ingredients to find the combinations you like best...

Our only 'rule' is that you ALWAYS include protein and/or good fats in your smoothie such as low-fat live natural yogurt, ground nuts, ground seeds, organic silken tofu, protein powder (try whey, pea or hemp), coconut milk or avocado. The protein and fat will slow the absorption of the juice into your blood stream, thereby preventing a blood glucose spike as well as keep you feeling fuller for longer. For extra 'oomph' add a scoop of protein powder to the recipes below.

Choose from: apple, apricot, avocado, banana, beetroot, blackberries, blueberries, broccoli, carrot, celeriac, celery, cherry, cucumber, fennel, ginger, grape, grapefruit, guava, kale, kiwi, lemon, lettuce, lime, mango, melon, mint, orange, papaya, parsley, passion fruit, peach, pear, pineapple, plum, raspberries, red pepper, spinach, strawberries, tomato, watercress, watermelon...

The thickness of a smoothie is very much down to personal choice so add a little water or coconut water if the smoothie is too thick for you.

Any leftover smoothie can be kept covered in the fridge for up to 48 hours.

Avocado Smoothie

Approx 4 servings

170g (6oz) seedless grapes
1 avocado, stoned, peeled and chopped
1 ripe pear, chopped
Juice of 1 lemon
Few drops tabasco, optional
4 almonds or 1 tsp almond butter, optional

Place the grapes, avocado, pear and almonds (if using) in a blender. Squeeze the juice from the lemon into the grape mix, with the tabasco if using. Blend everything together until smooth.

Berry Smoothie

Approx 4 servings

300g fresh or frozen strawberries, blueberries or raspberries
½ large avocado (about 100g), peeled
½ small cucumber (about 100g)
½ tin full fat coconut milk, about 200ml
12 almonds (preferably having been soaked in water overnight)

Wash the veg and fruit then blend everything together until smooth, adding water if needed to create your preferred consistency.

Green smoothie

Approx 4 servings

½ large cucumber, about 200g
1 apple, cored
1 stick celery
40g spinach or kale
½ large avocado (about 100g), peeled
Small handful watercress
1 inch piece fresh root ginger
Small handful fresh parsley
3 tablespoons lemon juice

Wash the fruit, veg and herbs then blend them with the rest of the ingredients until smooth. Add more water if needed to achieve your desired consistency.

Passion fruit, grape and banana

Approx 2 servings

1 ripe passion fruit, halved and pulp scooped out
40ml low-fat plain (natural) bio-live yogurt
1 small banana
55g (2oz) seedless grapes

Place all the ingredients in a blender and process until smooth. The passion fruit pips will stay whole but are easy to drink.

Beetroot Buzz

Approx 2-3 servings

100ml fresh apple juice
50ml fresh orange juice
50g cooked fresh beetroot
40ml low-fat plain (natural) bio-live yogurt
1" piece fresh root ginger
2 baby carrots

Place all the ingredients in your blender and whizz until smooth.

8.3 Broths

Bone broth

Makes approximately 3 litres

2-3kg bones – beef, lamb or chicken carcasses. Use saved bones from a roast or ask your butcher for unwanted bones.

A generous glug of apple cider vinegar or fresh lemon juice (this helps to extract minerals from the bones).

Place the bones into a large pan or slow cooker and cover with cold water. The water should cover the bones by a couple of inches. Add the apple cider vinegar or lemon juice.

Cover with a lid and bring to the boil. Reduce the heat and simmer gently with the lid on for at least 6 hours, skimming off any froth that rises to the top. The longer the bones simmer, the more nutrients are released.

Strain the liquid and cool before storing. The broth will keep in the fridge for several days or can be frozen in batches. Use in place of bought stock when making soup.

Vegetable broth

Makes approximately 3 litres

1 large onion, peeled and roughly chopped

1 large leek, thoroughly washed and roughly chopped

2 large carrots, roughly chopped

1 stalk celery, roughly chopped

3 garlic cloves, peeled and split with the flat of your knife

Fresh herbs – choose from parsley, thyme, tarragon, bay leaf

1 tsp sea salt
1 tsp black peppercorns
3 litres cold water

Put all the ingredients into a large pan and bring to a boil, then lower the heat and simmer for 45 minutes. Let the stock cool then strain into a clean container and discard the solids.

The stock will keep for a week in an airtight container in the fridge or can be frozen in batches. Use in place of bought stock when making soup.

8.4 *Smooth Soups*

Watercress and butter bean soup

Approx 8-12 servings

125g watercress, de-stalked
50g butter or coconut butter
200g leeks, cleaned and roughly chopped
1 tin butter beans
1 litre hot stock (homemade or Marigold Swiss vegetable bouillon powder)
2 heaped tablespoons of plain yogurt or fromage frais (optional)
Salt and freshly milled black pepper

Melt the butter in a pan and add the leek and some salt and cover the pan allowing the vegetables to sweat gently for about 20 minutes.

Add the stock and the beans and allow everything to simmer for another 10-15 minutes, adding the watercress one to two minutes before the end.

Allow to cool slightly and then blend (choosing how smooth you want it).

Stir through the yogurt if desired. This soup can also be served chilled.

Chickpea and leek soup

Approx 4-6 servings

½ cup dried chickpeas soaked overnight (or 1 tin)
1-3 leeks (depending on size)
1 small fennel bulb
Olive oil
1 clove of garlic (optional)
450 ml vegetable stock

Rinse the soaked chickpeas, cover with water and cook until tender.

Remove the outer skin of the leeks and slice finely. Slice the fennel bulb. Warm a thick-bottomed pan, add a good tablespoon of olive oil and gently sweat the leeks, fennel and garlic.

Add the drained chickpeas and the stock and simmer for 15 minutes. Season to taste.

The soup can be left chunky, liquidized or half liquidized. This soup is full of fibre and leeks are also a source of prebiotics.

Pumpkin and lentil soup

Approx 8-10 servings

1 cup of lentils (or a couple of tins)
1 small pumpkin or butternut squash
2 cloves of garlic
1 teaspoon of ground cumin
850 ml of vegetable or bone stock

Rinse the lentils (no need to soak), cover with water and cook until tender.

Remove the hard outer skin of the pumpkin/butternut squash and slice into chunks. Warm a thick-bottomed pan, add a good tablespoon of olive oil and add the pumpkin/butternut squash and cumin and sauté lightly for 5 minutes.

Add the drained lentils and the stock and simmer for 15-30 minutes until the pumpkin is cooked. This soup is best liquidised.

Easy Peasy Green soup

Approx 6-8 servings

2 tbsp coconut butter
1 medium onion, diced
300g frozen peas
2 bags watercress (organic if possible)
1-1/12 pints chicken stock (preferably homemade)
Sea salt and pepper

Sauté the onion in the coconut butter gently, until soft. Add the peas and stock and bring to the boil, then simmer for 5 minutes. Skim off any foam that comes to the surface. Add the watercress a minute or two before the end and then blend until smooth. Season to taste.

Roasted Mushroom Soup

Approx 6-8 servings

1kg mushrooms (ideally a mix of chestnut and open cap)
4 tablespoons coconut oil or ghee
4 garlic cloves, chopped
Leaves from small bunch flat-leaf parsley 650ml hot vegetable stock
Sea salt and freshly ground black pepper

Melt the oil in a large roasting tray. Remove stalks from the mushrooms then cut the caps in two quarters. Put caps and stalks in the roasting tray, ideally in one layer, season well and mix together. Roast for 25 minutes then stir in the garlic and return to the over for 5 more minutes.

Scrape the mushrooms and any juices from the roasting tray into a blender. Add most of the parsley leaves (reserving a few to garnish) and the stock and puree until smooth. Add a little more stock if required. Spoon into bowls and drizzle with extra virgin olive oil and sprinkle with reserved chopped parsley if you like.

Spicy Watercress and Broccoli Soup

Approx 4-6 servings

1 tbsp coconut oil
1 onion, chopped
4 cloves garlic, chopped
5cm piece fresh ginger, chopped
1 green chilli, deseeded (or more if preferred)
½ tsp cumin seeds
1 tsp fennel seeds
400ml vegetable stock
100g broccoli, roughly chopped
100g watercress

Melt the oil in a pan and sauté the onion gently and when soft add the garlic, chilli and spices and continue to cook for a couple of minutes.

Add the stock and bring to the boil. Add the broccoli and cook for a few minutes until it is bright green then add the watercress and let it wilt for a minute or two. Blend until smooth and season to taste.

Carrot, Coriander and Red Lentil Soup

Approx 8-10 servings

1kg carrots
120g red lentils
1 onion, chopped
1 litre vegetable stock
Good handful fresh coriander

Put all ingredients except the coriander in a pan and simmer for 45 minutes. Add the coriander and blend until smooth. Season to taste.

Vegetable soup

Approx 8-10 servings

This soup can be made with a wide range of vegetables, whatever you have in the fridge or freezer. It freezes well.

2 tablespoons olive or coconut oil
1 large onion, chopped or 1 thinly sliced leek
300ml vegetable stock (homemade or Marigold bouillon)
1 can chopped tomatoes, with juice
1 tbsp tomato purée
4 cups mixed fresh or frozen vegetables – choose from broccoli, carrots, corn, cauliflower, green beans, peas and courgettes (cut vegetables into similar sized pieces).
1 large stalk celery, sliced
2 tsp dried herbs – basil, oregano, mixed herbs
Coarse salt and ground pepper

Heat oil in a large pan over a medium heat. Add onions or leeks and cook, stirring frequently, until soft, 5 to 8 minutes.

Add stock, tomatoes and their juice and tomato purée and bring mixture to the boil. Reduce heat to a simmer, and cook, uncovered, for 20 minutes. Add vegetables and herbs to pan and return to a simmer. Cook, uncovered, until vegetables are tender, about 20 minutes. Season with salt and pepper, as desired, and blend to serve.

8.5 'Chunky' Soups

Thai style lentil and coconut soup

Approx 4-6 servings

2 tbsp coconut oil
2 red onions, finely chopped
1 bird's eye chilli, seeded and finely sliced
2 garlic cloves, chopped
1"/2.5cm piece fresh lemon grass, outer layers removed and inside finely sliced**
7oz/200g red lentils, rinsed
1 tsp/5mg ground coriander
1 tsp/5mg paprika
14 fl oz/400ml coconut milk
Juice of 1 lime
3 spring onions, chopped
¾ oz/20g fresh coriander, finely chopped salt and freshly ground black pepper

Heat the oil in a large pan and add the onions, chilli, garlic and lemon grass. Cook for 5 minutes or until the onions have softened but not browned, stirring occasionally.

Add the lentils and spices. Pour in the coconut milk and 1½ pints/900ml water and stir. Bring to the boil, reduce the heat and simmer for about 40 minutes, until the lentils are soft.

Pour in the lime juice and add the spring onions and coriander, reserving a little of each for the garnish. Season to taste, ladle into bowls, garnish and enjoy.

**Tip: Instead of fresh lemon grass, you can use ready-prepared paste which is sold in jars.

Leek and potato broth

Approx 8-10 servings

1 carrot, roughly sliced
1 stick celery, roughly sliced
1 medium onions, roughly chopped
200g leeks, thoroughly washed and sliced
1 clove garlic, peeled and sliced 100g potatoes, peeled and diced
Olive oil
1 litre chicken or vegetable stock
Sea salt freshly ground black pepper

Place a large pan on the heat and add 2 tablespoons of olive oil. Add all the prepared vegetables except the potatoes and mix together. Cook for about 10 minutes until the veg have softened slightly and are lightly golden.

Add the hot stock to the vegetables, along with the potatoes. Stir well and bring to the boil, then reduce the heat and simmer for 10 minutes with the lid on

Remove the pan from the heat and season with salt and pepper, to taste.

If you want this to be a light broth, remove the vegetables at this point and serve the broth. If you would prefer a thicker soup, liquidise about three quarters of the mix until smooth.

Mediterranean style soup

Approx 8-10 servings

1 large onion, chopped
2 sticks celery, chopped
1 red pepper, deseeded and chopped
2 cloves garlic, crushed
2 tbsp olive oil
2 tsps fresh oregano
1 tbsp tomato puree
2 x 390g cartons chopped tomatoes
200g dried red lentils
1 litre veg stock
1 x 400g tin chickpeas, drained and rinsed juice of 1 lemon
1 x 25g fresh basil, roughly chopped

Purée the onion, celery, red pepper and garlic in a food processor. Heat the olive oil gently in large pan and cook purée for about 5 mins.

Stir in oregano then add tomato puree, tomatoes and lentils along with the stock.

Bring to boil then simmer with lid on for 30 mins.

Uncover and add chickpeas, cook for further 5 mins, topping up with water if necessary. Season to taste. Stir through lemon juice and chopped coriander just before serving.

Spicy Lentil and Chickpea Soup

Approx 8-10 servings

A delicious, filling and wholesome meal of a soup that tastes even better the next day.

1 tbsp butter or coconut butter
1 onion, chopped
1 clove garlic, crushed
1 (14 oz) can whole tomatoes or passata
2 tbsp fresh chopped coriander
$\frac{1}{4}$ tsp ground ginger
$\frac{1}{2}$ tsp cinnamon
$\frac{1}{2}$ tsp turmeric
$\frac{1}{2}$ tsp ground cumin
1 cup (8 oz) red lentils, rinsed
4 cups (850ml) water or miso
14 oz can organic chickpeas, drained
$\frac{1}{2}$ tsp sea salt
$\frac{1}{4}$ tsp ground black pepper

Heat the butter in a large pan over a medium heat. Add the onions and garlic and cook gently until they soften, stirring occasionally – about 5 minutes.

Meanwhile, blend the tomatoes in a food processor until smooth or use passata if preferred.

Add the spices and coriander to the onions and cook for one minute. Add the tomato mixture and bring to a boil. Add the lentils and water (or miso if preferred), cover and reduce heat to low and simmer until the lentils are tender – about 20 minutes.

Add the chickpeas and raise the heat, until simmering, for about 10 minutes then serve.

Tomato, Carrot and Lentil Soup

Approx 5 servings

1 large onion, chopped
200g can tomatoes
2 medium carrots, grated
500ml water or stock
2 tsp tomato puree
75g red split lentils
1 bay leaf
1 tsp turmeric
1 heaped tsp cumin
Sea salt and freshly ground black pepper to taste

Soften the onions, tomatoes and carrots in the stock with the tomato puree, bay leaf, turmeric and cumin for 5 minutes over a gentle heat. Add the lentils, cover and bring to the boil. Turn down the heat and simmer gently for 40 minutes. Season to taste.

Serve chunky or liquidise, whichever you prefer.

Moroccan spiced soup

Approx 8-10 servings

1 large onion, chopped
2 sticks celery, chopped
1 red pepper, deseeded and chopped
2 cloves garlic, crushed
2 tbsp olive oil
1 stick cinnamon
1 tsp ground coriander
1 tsp smoked paprika
1 tsp ground chilli
1 tbsp tomato puree
2 tsp xylitol or honey
2 x 390g cartons chopped tomatoes
200g dried red lentils
1 litre vegetable stock
1 x 400g tin chickpeas, drained and rinsed
Juice of 1 lemon
1x 25g pack fresh coriander, roughly chopped

In a food processor, blend the onion, celery, red pepper and garlic to a puree. Heat the oil in a large pan and cook the puree for about 5 minutes.

Stir in the cinnamon stick, ground coriander, paprika and chilli. Cook for about 1 minute, until fragrant, then stir in the tomato puree and sugar. Add the chopped tomatoes and lentils to the pan along with the stock.

Bring to the boil then simmer with the lid on for 30 minutes. Uncover and add the chickpeas, cook for a further 5 minutes, topping up with water if necessary. Season to taste. Stir through the lemon juice and chopped coriander just before serving.

Tip: Try adding some fresh or frozen spinach just before serving.

8.6 Breakfast Ideas

Protein packed breakfast

Approx 2 servings

2 heaped tbsp mixed seeds – sunflower, sesame, pumpkin, chia, flaxseed
1 tbsp whole almonds, roughly chopped (optional)
1 dessert spoon coconut oil
Coconut milk, fresh pineapple juice or fresh apple juice
1 apple, pear, banana or plum or a handful fresh berries – raspberries, blueberries and/or blackberries

Before you go to bed cover the seeds and nuts (if using) in the juice or coconut milk.

In the morning simply stir in the coconut oil and grate the apple and/or pear or chop the banana or plum in to the seed mix. Add a little more coconut milk or juice to your preferred consistency and top with a few fresh berries. A great way to start the day!

NB: Soaking the nuts and seeds overnight neutralises the phytic acid in them, greatly helping their digestion and absorption. A tablespoon of gluten free oats could be soaked overnight with the seeds for a bigger breakfast.

Warm and wholesome porridge

Approx 1 serving

50g (2oz) whole porridge oats
250ml water
½ an apple, grated
1 tbsp mixed ground seeds (sunflower, pumpkin and flaxseeds)
½ tsp ground cinnamon

In a saucepan, bring the oats and water to the boil and then gently simmer for a few minutes, until cooked. Just before serving, add the grated apple and cinnamon and stir well. Serve, sprinkling the ground seeds over the top.

Substitute the apple with pear and a handful of blueberries if preferred.

3. Omelette

Filled with choice of diced pepper, tomatoes, mushroom, cheese, ham, smoked salmon and chives, or a sprinkling of dried herbs.

4. Scrambled eggs

With a choice of mushrooms, onions, peppers, tomatoes or smoked salmon.

Apple, almond and cinnamon pancakes

Approx 3 servings

1½ cups almond powder/flour
3 eggs
1 cup water/milk
1 apple grated
½ teaspoon cinnamon powder

Crack the eggs into a bowl and whisk, add the rest of the ingredients and mix to a batter like consistency.

Heat a frying pan and add a few drops of oil. Do not let it smoke.

Add a ladle of batter and cook the pancakes for 2-3minutes on each side until golden brown.

This makes about 8 small pancakes.

8.7 *Meals*

Cod, chorizo and chickpea stew

Approx 4-6 servings

1 tbsp olive oil
1 onion, chopped
100g chorizo sausage, skinned and chopped
1 red or yellow pepper, sliced
1 clove garlic, crushed
½ tsp sweet smoked paprika
½ fish or veg stock cube
A pinch of saffron
1 x 400g tin chopped tomatoes
1 x 400g tin chickpeas, drained
About 350g cod loin, cut into large chunks
Chopped parsley to serve

Heat the olive oil in a large saucepan and cook the onions gently for about 10 minutes, until soft. Add the chorizo and cook for a further 5 minutes, then add the peppers, garlic and paprika and cook for 3-4 minutes.

Meanwhile, stir the stock cube and saffron into 200ml boiling water. Pour into the chorizo mixture and add the tomatoes and chickpeas. Stir, season with salt and freshly ground black pepper, then cover and cook for 10 minutes.

Place the pieces of cod on top of the stew, then cover and cook for 8-10 minutes.

Serve sprinkled with the parsley and a mound of freshly steamed vegetables.

Salmon with soy, ginger and spring onion

1 salmon fillet
1 tbsp orange juice
½ tbsp soy sauce
1-2 spring onions, very finely sliced
1 tsp grated fresh root ginger

Place the salmon fillet on a square of greaseproof paper in a square of foil large enough to form a loose parcel.

Mix the orange juice, soy sauce and ginger in a bowl. Scatter two thirds of the spring onion over the fish. Pour the juice mixture over the fish and fold the paper/foil loosely to form a parcel. Leave to stand for at least 10 minutes to allow the flavours to mingle.

Cook in the oven at 150 degrees C, 300 F, gas 2 for 10-15 minutes, until the fish is cooked. Serve with the juices from the parcel and the rest of the spring onion scattered over the fish. Ideal served with stir fried mixed vegetables.

Salmon and haddock kebab with coriander and sunflower pesto

Approx 3-4 servings

100g piece skinless haddock fillet (or other white fish)
100g skinless salmon fillet
Juice of 1/2 lime
1 tsp extra virgin olive oil
Freshly ground pepper (to taste)
50g brown rice or quinoa
For the pesto:
A bunch of fresh coriander (25g)
25g sunflower seeds
1 clove garlic, peeled
1 tbsp olive oil

Cut the fish into large chunks and thread onto skewers. Mix the lime juice, oil and black pepper and pour evenly over the kebabs. Leave to stand until required for cooking.

Cook the rice or quinoa.

To make the pesto, place the coriander, sunflower seeds and garlic in a food processor and process quickly. Do not allow the mixture to get too fine. Moisten with the olive oil and keep to one side.

Place the kebabs under a hot grill for 2-3 minutes each side until just cooked through. Do not allow the fish to overcook or it will be hard and unpleasant. Serve with the rice/quinoa and pesto.

Roast fish with herbs and tomatoes

Serves 1

1 fillet of cod or haddock per person
Olive oil
½ a large tomato per fillet, sliced
A generous handful of fresh herbs (rosemary and thyme)
Some lemon zest
A squeeze of lemon juice

Brush each fish fillet with olive oil and cover each fillet with sliced tomato. Crush the herbs a little so they release their fragrance and place on top of the fish. Add the lemon zest, a squeeze of lemon juice and season with salt and ground black pepper.

Wrap the fish in greaseproof paper and then in foil to form a loose parcel. Roast at 190 °C, gas mark 5, for 15 minutes.

Serve with the herby olive oil that's puddled around the fish and some steamed vegetables or a mixed salad.

Grilled chicken with celeriac mash

Approx 3 servings

2 small chicken breast fillets, skinned
1 tablespoon flour
1 small egg, beaten
5-6 tablespoons sesame seeds
150 g (5 ½ oz) green beans, trimmed
Celeriac mash:
1 small celeriac
A little sea salt and freshly ground black pepper (to taste)

Cut the chicken fillets into two or three pieces. Coat very lightly with flour, dip in beaten egg and then dip in the sesame seeds. Make sure they are well coated.

Peel and slice the celeriac and cook in a steamer until tender. Then either place in a blender and purée or mash with a potato masher, adding salt and pepper to taste.

Place the coated chicken fillets in the grill pan under a hot grill and cook for about 5 minutes on each side until thoroughly cooked. Take care not to have the chicken too close to the heat or the seeds will burn.

Meanwhile, cook the green beans in a steamer or in a little water until they are *al dente* or still slightly crisp to the bite. Serve with the sesame grilled chicken and celeriac mash.

Chicken with Rosemary

Approx 6 servings

1 tbsp oil
75g pancetta cubes
6 spring onions, sliced
1 small clove garlic, chopped
1 tsp fresh rosemary, finely chopped
500g boneless skinless chicken thighs, cut into bite-sized pieces
½ tsp celery salt (or sea salt)
125ml white wine (or replace with extra stock if preferred)
½ pint chicken stock
2 bay leaves
1 x 400g tin cannellini beans, rinsed and drained (or use any other pulse of choice)

Heat the oil in a pan and gently fry the pancetta, spring onions, garlic and rosemary for 2-3 minutes. Add the chicken pieces and salt and stir well.

Pour in the wine, if using, and bring to a simmer, then add the stock, bay leaves, xylitol or honey and beans. Cover with a lid and leave to simmer for 15 minutes or until the beans are warmed through and the chicken is cooked. Serve with freshly steamed vegetables.

Moroccan chicken with apricots and lemon

Approx 3 servings

1 tbsp Moroccan spice mix
2½ tbsp vegetable oil
4 skin-on chicken thighs
8 ready-to-eat apricots (or pitted prunes, if you prefer)
1 small lemon, cut into 8 wedges
200g barley couscous
3 tbsp frozen petits pois
250ml hot vegetable stock
1 tsp butter
1 x 150ml pot natural yogurt

Mix the spice mix with 2 tbsp of oil and a pinch of salt and rub into the chicken thighs.

Heat the remaining oil in a large frying pan. Add the chicken thighs skin side down and brown over a high heat. Turn the chicken over and scatter the apricots and lemon wedges on top. Cover and cook over a medium heat for 20 minutes, turning halfway through.

Shortly before serving, mix the couscous with the frozen peas in a bowl. Add the hot stock, stir, then cover and leave for 5 minutes. Stir in the butter, season and fluff with a fork.

Serve the chicken, apricots and lemon with the couscous and some yogurt.

Chicken and lentil curry

Approx 5 servings

500g skinless chicken thigh fillets, each cut into 6
1 tbsp sunflower oil
2 medium onions, peeled and roughly chopped
1½ tbsp medium curry powder
100g dried red lentils, rinsed
400ml chicken stock
250g basmati rice
150g spinach
125g low-fat natural yogurt

Season the chicken. Heat the oil in a casserole, add the chicken and fry for 5 minutes. Add the onions and fry for 3 minutes, stirring. Reduce the heat slightly, stir in the curry powder and cook for 1 minute to release the flavour. Add the lentils and stock, cover and simmer for 15 minutes or until the lentils are tender.

Meanwhile, cook the rice. Just before it's ready, check the seasoning of the curry, stir in the spinach leaves and cook until just beginning to wilt (about 2 minutes). Swirl in the yogurt and serve the curry with the rice.

8.8 Snack Ideas

Tasty Carrot Salad

1 serving

This tasty salad is great as a healthy snack or side salad.
1 medium carrot, grated
handful fresh coriander, stems removed
2 tsp sesame seeds
small knob of fresh ginger root
1 tbsp extra virgin olive oil
dash of soy sauce or tamari
pepper

Grate the carrot into a bowl and add the chopped coriander, finely grated ginger and sesame seeds. Pour over the olive oil and soy sauce and season with the pepper (no salt as the soy will be salty enough). Mix everything thoroughly and enjoy.

Kale Crisps

Multiple servings

Large head of kale
Knob of coconut oil or ghee
Sea salt

Preheat oven to 100°C. Place baking sheet with the oil in the oven to warm.

Remove the stalks from the kale and tear the greens roughly.

Toss the kale in the oil and bake for 10 minutes. Turn the kale over, add a little salt and return to the oven. Keep an eye on it as it can burn quickly and will taste bitter.

Once crispy remove and serve. Can be stored in an airtight container.

Super-Quick Courgette salad

1 serving

Alkalising and tasty, this salad is quick to make and can be used as a snack or side salad.
1 courgette
A handful of pumpkin seeds
1 tbsp extra virgin olive oil 2 tsp balsamic vinegar
Sea salt and black pepper

Toast the pumpkin seeds in a dry frying pan over a medium heat. Watch the seeds all the time as they burn really easily. Shake the pan every minute, until the seeds are golden and start to jump around.

Wash the courgette, dry it and grate into a bowl. Sprinkle the seeds over the courgette and drizzle over the oil and vinegar and season with the salt and pepper. Eat straight away. If making this in advance, keep the grated courgette covered and only add the dressing just before eating.

Savoury flapjacks

Multiple servings

An alternative to the usual sweet snack.
200g Pecorino cheese, cut in 3 cm chunks
1 small handful fresh basil or parsley, leaves only
150g onion, peeled and very finely chopped
200g carrots, peeled if not organic, grated
200g courgettes, grated
200g jumbo oats **or** gluten-free oats
2 large eggs

Preheat the oven to 190°C/375°F/gas mark 5 and line the base of a shallow, square 20cm x 20cm baking tin with greaseproof paper.

Grate the cheese together with the fresh herbs. Add the onion, carrots and courgettes and mix well. Add the oats followed by the eggs and mix well. Place mixture into the prepared baking tin and bake for 25 to 30 minutes until golden brown.

Remove from the oven and cut into pieces then leave to cool in the tin before removing.

Chilli and Rosemary Seed Bars

Multiple servings

A great alternative to the usual sweet snack. Quinoa flakes and rice malt syrup should be available from health food shops.

125g quinoa flakes
50ml coconut oil (aroma free) or rapeseed oil
300g pumpkin seeds
125g sunflower seeds
1 tablespoon finely chopped fresh rosemary
¼ tsp salt
½ tsp dried chilli flakes, or to taste
200g rice malt syrup

Preheat oven to 170°C/Gas 3. Line a 19-20cm square baking dish with greaseproof paper.

Put quinoa flakes in a large dry frying pan over a medium heat and toast for a couple of minutes, tossing or stirring them often. When they look and smell toasty, but barely coloured, tip them into a large bowl.

Add pumpkin seeds to the pan and slightly increase the heat. Cook, stirring, for about 3 minutes or until the seeds are lightly golden then tip them into the bowl with the quinoa. Then add the sunflower seeds to the pan, cooking and stirring until nicely coloured, add to the bowl with the pumpkin seeds.

Mix the rosemary, salt and chilli flakes in to the mixture.

Put the coconut oil and rice malt syrup in the pan and heat gently until it just starts to simmer. Add to the seeds and mix everything together well. Scrape mixture into the lined baking dish, press it into an even layer and bake for 15 minutes or until just golden on top.

Allow to cool completely in the dish then lift the greaseproof paper out and cut into bars. Store in an airtight container. They keep well for several weeks.

Spicy hummus

Multiple servings

Hummus is a rich spread that is full of protein. It can be used as a snack on oatcakes or eaten with raw vegetables (carrot, celery, cucumber, tomatoes, peppers and broccoli) or as a satisfying lunch in a filled wholemeal pitta bread or 'wrap' with salad.

1½ cups raw organic chickpeas (tinned, preferably organic, may also be used)
1 tbsp vegetable oil
3 cloves garlic, crushed
1 dessertspoon tamari or soy sauce
¾ cup tahini
¼ cup finely chopped parsley (or coriander)
¼ cup finely chopped spring onions
Juice from 1 lemon
Black and cayenne pepper to taste
½ tsp sea salt

Soak chickpeas overnight and boil until very soft (1 1/2 hours), then blend to a thick paste, using a food processor. Combine all other ingredients and chill thoroughly. Serve as above.

Substitutions
- The chickpeas can be substituted with any type of bean or pea processed the same way – such as red kidney beans, butter beans, split green peas, etc.
- Any nut or seed butter can be used instead of tahini – try almond, sesame, peanut or pumpkin butter.

Chopped coriander or roasted red peppers may also be added for flavour and variety.

Chapter 9

Checklists

Checklists for Gastric Band Wearers

We have provided these checklists as an overview for the gastric band wearer. This list is not exhaustive and we recommend that you personalise and update them where appropriate. Please keep your records.

1) Medications associated with body fat and weight gain

2) Biochemical Tests and Micro Nutrient Analysis

3) Common Deficiencies

4) Minimum supplement plan

5) Follow-up appointments

6) Pregnancy after weight-loss surgery

7) Members of your healthcare and wellness team?

8) In the kitchen

9.1 Medications associated with body fat and weight gain

Medication Class and subtype	Medication Drug	Yes/No/Not applicable Prior to surgery	Yes/No/Not applicable Post surgery
Psychiatric or neurologic agents			
Antipsychotic agents	Phenothiazines, olanzapine, clozapine, risperidone		
Mood stabilizers	Lithium		
Antidepressants	Tricyclics, MAOIs monoamine oxidase inhibitors, SSRIs, selective serotonin reuptake inhibitors. mirtazapine		
Antiepileptic drugs	Gabapentin, valproate, carbamazepine		
Steroid hormones			
Corticosteroids	-		
Progestational steroids	-		
Antidiabetes agents	Insulin, sulfonylureas, thiazolidinediones		
Antihypertensive agents	Beta-Adrenergic and Alpha-adrenergic receptor blockers		
Antihistamines	Cyproheptadine		
HIV protease inhibitors			

Mechanick et al., (2009) AACE/TOS/ASMBS Guidelines.

9.2 Biochemical Tests and Micro Nutrient Analysis

General and Nutritional	Pre-surgery Date:	Post-surgery Date:	Post-surgery Date:	Post-surgery Date:	Post-surgery Date:	Post-surgery Date:
BOMSS recommendations (if not following nutritionally balanced diet):						
Full blood count	*	**				
Ferritin	*					
Folate	*					
Vitamin B12	*					
25 hydroxy-vitamin D	*	**?				
Calcium	*					
Parathyroid hormone	*					
Liver function test	*	**				
Urea and electrolytes	*	**				
Comorbidities						
Fasting Glucose	*					
HbA1c	*	**?				
Lipid profile	*	**?				
ASMBS also recommend…						
Homocysteine						
Vitamin A						
Vitamin E (optional)						

Bone density (at 2 years)					
We also suggest…					
Full nutrient screen					
Digestive screen					
Additional personalised tests depending on your circumstances (adrenal, bone turnover, hormones, food allergy, genetics etc.)					
Veyrune et al., (2008) also recommend…					
Full dental check inc. chewing ability.					

* = The British Obesity and Metabolic Surgery Society recommend all of the above prior to any type of bariatric surgery (Kane et al., 2014).

** = For follow-ups

**? = For follow-ups where required

9.3 Common Deficiencies

Common deficiencies found in obese individuals, candidates prior to weight-loss surgery, and then following gastric banding. These are unlikely to improve after surgery without due care and attention.

Biomarker	Obese or pre-op	Gastric band wearer
Protein		↓
Iron	↓ 43.9% (more common in younger patients)	↓ 30-57% iron-deficiency anaemia rising to 72% after 18 months
Ferritin	↓ 8.4% (more common in women)	↓
Haemoglobin	↓ 22%	↓
Thiamine	↓ 29%	↓ Common
Vitamin D	↓ 25-80%	↓
Vitamin A	↓ 12.5%	↓
B12	↓ 3.5%	↓
Meet criteria for hyperparathyroidism	23.5%	
Selenium	↓	↓
Chromium	↓	↓
B6	↓ Lower than in healthy weight people	↓
Vitamin C	↓ Lower than in healthy weight people	↓ Up to 35%
Vitamin E	↓ Lower than in healthy weight people	↓
Zinc	↓ Around 28%	↓

Full descriptions and references can be found in Chapter 6.

9.4 Minimum Supplement Plan

Supplement	Adult	Yes/Not applicable and why
Routine Supplements		
Multi vitamin and mineral including iron, folate and thiamine	1 daily	
Elemental calcium (in diet and as calcium citrate supplement in divided doses)	1,200 – 1,500 mg/day	
Vitamin D	3000 IU/day	
Vitamin B12	As needed to maintain normal levels	
Personalised supplements (where appropriate)		
Protein Powders		
Essential Fatty Acids		
Liver Support		
Pre & Probiotics		
Other		
1)		
2)		
3)		
4)		
5)		

Patients with pre or postoperative biochemical deficiencies should have a personalised supplement plan beyond these recommendations. Full descriptions and references can be found in Chapter 8.

Adapted from: Mechanick et al., (2013) AMSBS [http://asmbs.org/wp/uploads/2014/05/AACE_TOS _ASMBS_Clinical_Practice_Guidli nes_3.2013.pdf]

9.5 Follow-up Appointments

Nutritional or metabolic co-morbidities → **YES** → Every month as circumstances require for first 6 months → 6-12 months **TWICE** → 12 – 24 months **TWICE** (every six months) → Onwards **ANNUALLY**

Nutritional or metabolic co-morbidities → **NO** → Every month as circumstances require for first 6 months → 6-12 months **ONCE** → 12 – 24 months **ONCE** → Onwards **ANNUALLY**

We recommend you speak with your bariatric team to find out exactly how many follow-up appointments you will have access to, and specifically what and who they will include.

Adapted from: Mechanick et al., (2009) AACE/TOS/ASMBS Guidelines.

9.6 Pregnancy after weight-loss surgery

*** Important – Please read Chapter 6 and 7 regarding alternatives to folic acid supplementation.

Recommendation	Adult	Yes/No/ Not applic.	Appt. 1 Prenatal	Appt. 2 First Trimester	Appt. 3 Second Trimester	Appt. 4 Third Trimester
Reliable contraception for 12 – 24 months after surgery						
Prenatal Multi-vitamin – 1a-day to include vitamin A as a natural beta carotene, zinc (15mg) copper (2mg), iodine (100-150mg) and magnesium						
Folic Acid*** - 400mcg daily - replace with additional doses if deficiency has been confirmed.						
Vitamin D3 – 2,000- 6,000IU/day depending on status						
Calcium citrate – 1500mg daily (take 2hrs away from multivitamin)						
Elemental Iron (4065mg/day)						
Vitamin B12 350μg/day orally, replace with additional doses if deficiency has been confirmed						
Regular lab tests						
Regular ultrasound scans follow up which evaluates foetal growth and mineralization of skeleton.						
Close follow up of weight changes during pregnancy and postpartum.						

(Kominiarrek et al., 2011, Kaska et al., 2013, Mechanick et al., 2013)

9.7 *Your healthcare and wellness team*

You may have a few people or more —feel free to adapt and add to this list.

Who	Contact details	Yes/No/ Not applicable	What they offer?
Bariatric specialists			
Bariatric Surgeon			
Bariatric Coordinator (e.g. advanced practice nurse)			
RD/Nutritionist/Registered NT			
Medical Consultants			
Psychologist or psychiatrist			
Endocrinologist			
Physician nutrition specialist			
Certified nutrition support clinician			
Sleep medicine specialist			
Cardiologist			
Gastroenterologist			
Psychiatrist			
Support personnel			
Hospital/surgery support group			
Cosmetic surgeon			
Movement specialist			
NLP, CBT, Hypnotherapy			
Holistic (such as reiki, massage, yoga therapy, tai-chi, talking therapies, flower remedies, aromatherapy, meditation teachers).			
Family and friends			

Adapted from:

Mechanick et al., (2009) AACE/TOS/ASMBS Guidelines.

9.8 In the Kitchen

Bariatric surgery is not only "life-changing" but also requires "changing one's life".

Nadia Ahmed, Director of Obesity Medical Institute, Dubai

The changes that individuals need to go through after surgery is quite phenomenal, here we have focused on the kitchen. Being organised and learning new skills is an essential part of your journey to success.

Item	Yes/No/ Not applicable	Pre surgery	Post surgery
Equipment			
Slow cooker			
Blender			
Juicer			
Decent knife			
Decent peeler			
Decent chopping board			
Small glass containers to chill or freeze portions of food			
Jam jars for smoothies/juices			
Produce			
Fresh fruits			
Fresh vegetables			
Whole grains			
Good quality protein (meat, fish, eggs, beans, pulses, tofu, protein powders)			
Skills			
Learn about food			
Learn how to cook			
Learn how to uncook (i.e. raw foods – quick and easy)			
Be prepared			
New ways of living take time			
Allocate time			
Be kind to yourself and enjoy the journey			

Summary:

✓ Check medications that may be contributing to your weight gain

✓ Ensure you have basic biochemical tests and additional tests if indicated

✓ Check common deficiencies alongside signs and symptoms discussed in Chapter 6 and note which may apply to you.

✓ Follow the minimum supplement plan – or your personalised plan

✓ Ensure you attend routine and follow up appointments

✓ If you are considering conceiving or are pregnant use the pregnancy after weight-loss surgery checklist

✓ Note contact details of your healthcare and wellness team

✓ Consider what changes you need to make in the kitchen

> *Watch with glittery eyes the whole world around you because the greatest secrets are always hidden in the most unlikely places.*
>
> Roald Dahl

We hope you have found this information useful and wish you the best of luck with your weight-loss journey whether this be with or without a band.

Chapter 10

Moving Forward

10.1 What is Nutritional Therapy?

Nutritional therapy is a process-based assessment of individual drivers of health, which facilitates a truly personalised approach to nutrition, diet and lifestyle recommendations. Developed in the United States as 'functional medicine', it is practised in the UK by nutritional therapy practitioners and in the US by functional medicine dieticians.

The basis of Nutritional Therapy

Nutritional Therapy is the application of nutrition science in the promotion of health, peak performance and individual care. Nutritional therapy practitioners use a wide range of tools to assess and identify potential nutritional imbalances and understand how these may contribute to an individual's symptoms and health concerns. This approach allows them to work with individuals to address nutritional balance and help support the body towards maintaining health.

Nutritional therapy is recognised as a complementary medicine and is relevant for individuals with chronic conditions, as well as those looking for support to enhance their health and wellbeing.

Practitioners consider each individual to be unique and recommend personalised nutrition and lifestyle programmes rather than a 'one size fits all' approach. Practitioners never recommend nutritional therapy as a replacement for medical advice and always refer any client with 'red flag' signs or symptoms to their medical professional. They will also frequently work alongside a medical professional and will communicate with other healthcare professionals involved in the client's care to explain any nutritional therapy programme that has been provided.

10.2 Choosing a Practitioner

Training:

It is important to choose a qualified Registered Nutritional Therapist who has undertaken all the necessary training to understand the theory and practice of nutritional therapy. For more information follow the link:

www.cnhcregister.org.uk/newsearch/index.cfm

Voluntary Regulation:

By choosing Nutritional Therapists registered with the CNHC you can be confident that they are properly trained, qualified and insured.

Professional Association:

By choosing a Registered Nutritional Therapist who is a member of BANT you can be confident that they follow the strict CNHC Code of Conduct, Performance and Ethics and the BANT Professional Practice Handbook, have professional indemnity insurance for clinical practice and also meet the membership entry criteria found at this link:

www.bant.org.uk/nutritional-therapy-careers/join-bant/apply-formembership/full-membership/

References

Aasheim E, Hofsø D, Hjelmesæth J, Birkelan Kd, Bøhmer T (2008) Vitamin status in morbidly obese patients: a cross-sectional study. *American Society for Clinical Nutrition,* **87**:2:362-369.

Aasheim E, Bjorkman S, Sovik T, Engstrom M, Hanvold S, Mala T Olbers T, Bøhmer T (2009) Vitamin status after bariatric surgery: a randomized study of gastric bypass and duodenal switch. *American Journal of Clinical Nutrition,* **90**:15–22.

Adams & Hewison (2010) Update in Vitamin D. *Journal of Clinical Endocrinology and Metabolism,* **95**:2: 471–478.

Ahima (2006) Adipose Tissue and Endocrine Organ. *Obesity,* **14**:S242- S248.

Alatishe A, Ammori BJ, Syed AA (2012) Pregnancy after bariatric surgery does not affect weight loss. *British Medical Journal* **345**:e6293.

Alberta Health Care Services (2013) *Nutrition Guideline: Bariatric Surgery for Adults.* Available at: [http://www.albertahealthservices.ca/hp/if-hp-ed-cdm-ns-5-6-3-bariatric-surgery-for-adults.pdf]. Accessed: 20th November 2014.

American College of Obstetricians and Gynecologists (2013) Obesity in pregnancy. Committee Opinion No. 549. *Obstetrics and Gynecology,* **121**:1:213-7.

American College of Obstetricians and Gynecologists (2013) Weight gain during pregnancy. Committee Opinion No. 548. *Obstetrics and Gynecology,* **121**:210–2.

Appelhans B, Whited M, Schneider K, Ma Y, Oleski J, Merriam P, Waring M, Olendzki B, Mann D, Ockene I, Pagot S (2012) Depression Severity, Diet Quality and Physical Activity in Women with Obesity and Depression. *Journal of the Academy of Nutrition and Dietetics,* **112**:5: 693-698.

Attar & Bowman (2014) Rising Threat of Environmental Toxins, Link to Chronic Diseases. *American Nurse* **46**:2.

Baboota R, Bishnoi M, Ambalam P, Kondepudi K, Sarma S, Bopari R, Podili K (2013) Functional food ingredients for the management of obesity and associated co-morbidities – A review. *Journal of Functional Foods* **5**:997-1012.

Bailey R, Looker A, Gahche J, Mills J, Weaver C (2014) Homocysteine and bone mineral density in older females in the United States (257.5) *The FASEB Journal,* **28**:1:257.5.

Baltaci D, Kutlucan A, Turker Y, Yilmaz A, Karacam S, Deler H, Ucgun T, Kara I (2013) Association of vitamin B12 with obesity, overweight, insulin resistance and metabolic syndrome, and body fat composition; primary care-based study. *Med Glas (Zenica)* **10**:2:203-10.

Bar-Zohar D, Azem F, Klausner J, Abu-Abeid S (2006) Pregnancy after laparoscopic adjustable gastric banding: perinatal outcome is favourable also for women with relatively high gestational weight gain. *Surgical Endoscopy*, **10**:1580-1583.

Bays (2009) Sick Fat, Metabolic Disease and Atherosclerosis. *The American Journal of Cardiology*, **122**:1:S26-S37.

Beccuti G, Pannain S (2011) Sleep and obesity. *Current opinion in clinical nutrition and metabolic care*, **14**(4):402-412.

Bendtsen LQ, Lorenzen JK, Bendsen NT, Rasmussen C, Astrup A (2013) Effect of Dairy Proteins on Appetite, Energy Expenditure, Body Weight, and Composition: a Review of the Evidence from Controlled Clinical Trials. *Advances in Nutrition*, **4**: 418-438.

Benelam B, Wyness L (2010) Hydration and health: a review. *British Nutrition Foundation Nutrition Bulletin*, **35**, 3–25.

Bennett W, Gilson M, Jamshidi R, Burke A, Segal K, Makary M, Clark J (2010) Impact of Bariatric Surgery on hypertensive disorders: retrospective analysis of insurance claim data. *British Medical Journal*, **340**: c1662.

Bernaert N, De Paepeb D, Boutene C, De Clercqb H, Stewartc D, Van Bockstaelea E, De Looseb M, Van Droogenbroeck B (2012) Antioxidant capacity, total phenolic and ascorbate content as a function of the genetic diversity of leek (Allium ampeloprasum var. porrum). *Food Chemistry*, **134**:2:669–677.

Bertoia, M, Pai J, Cooke J, Joosten, M, Mittleman M, Rimm E, Mukamal K (2014) Plasma homocysteine, dietary B vitamins, betaine, and choline and risk of peripheral artery disease. *Atherosclerosis*. Article in Press.

Bes-Rastrollo, Schulze M, Ruiz-Canela M, Martinez-Gonzalez M (2013) Financial Conflicts of Interest and Reporting Bias Regarding the Association between Sugar-Sweetened Beverages and Weight Gain: A Systematic Review of Systematic Reviews. *Plos medicine*. DOI: *10.1371/journal.pmed.1001578*. Available at: [http://www.plosmedicine.org/article/info%3Adoi%2F10.1371%2Fjournal.pmed.1001578]. Accessed: 4th December 2014.

Blair S, Diehl P, Massarini M, Sarto P, Sallis R, Searle J (2011) *Exercise is Medicine: A Quick Guide to Exercise Prescription*. TechnoGym: An Iniitiaive of the American College of Sports Nutrition.

Bond D, Wing R, Vithiananthan S, Sax H, Roye G, Ryder B, Pohl D, Giovanni J (2011) Significant resolution of female sexual dysfunction after bariatric surgery. *Surgery for Obesity and Related Diseases*, **7**:1:1–7.

Bonet L, Canas J, Ribot J, Palou A (2015) Carotenoids and their conversion products in the control of adipocyte function, adiposity and obesity. *Archives of Biochemistry and Biophysics*. **572**:112-125.

Boo & Harding (2006) The developmental origins of adult disease (Barker) Hypothesis. *Australian and New Zealand Journal of Obstetrics and Gynaecology*, **46**:4-14.

Bradley D, Conte C, Mittendorfer B, Eagon JC, VarelaJE, Fabbrini E eta al., (2012) Gastric bypass and banding equally improve insulin sensitivity and beta cell function. *Journal of Clinical Investigation.* **122**:12:4667-4674.

Brock K, Huang W, Fraser D, Ke L, Tseng M, Stolzenberg-Solomon R, Peters U, Ahn J, Purdue M, Mason R, McCarty C, Ziegler R, Graubard B (2010) Low Vitamin D status is associated with physical inactivity, obesity and low vitamin D intake in a large US sample of healthy middle aged men and women. *Journal of Steroid Biochemical Molecular Biology,* **121**:1-2: 462–466.

Brownley A, Boettiger C, Young L, Cefalu W (2015) Dietary chromium supplementation for targeted treatment of diabetes patients with comorbid depression and binge eating. *Medical Hypotheses* Article in Press. doi:10.1016/j.mehy.2015.03.020.

Brownley K, Von Holle A, Hamer R, La Via M, Bulik C (2013) A double-blind, randomized pilot trial of chromium picolinate for binge eating disorder: results of the Binge Eating and Chromium (BEACh) study. *Journal of Psychosomatic Research* **1**:75:36–42.

Brzozowska M, Sainsbury A, Eisman J, Baldock P, Center J (2014) Bariatric Surgery and Bone Loss: Do We Need to Be Concerned? *Clinical Reviews in Bone and Mineral Metabolism* **12**:4:207-227.

Buchwald H (2005) Bariatric surgery for morbid obesity: Health implications for patients, health professionals and third-party payers. *Surgery for Obesity and Related Diseases*, **1**: 371-381.

Cao J (2011) Effects of obesity on bone metabolism. *Journal of Orthopaedic Surgery and Research*, **6**:30.

Canon & Nedergaard, 2012 Neither Brown nor White. *Nature* **1**:7411:6-7.

Cartwright M, Wardle J, Steggles N, Simon A, Croker H; Jarvis M (2003) Stress and dietary practices in adolescents. *Health Psychology*, **22**:4:362-369.

Center For Alternative Medicine

[http://www.centerforaltmed.com/?page_id=8]. Accessed: 13th May 2015.

Chagas C, Saunders C, Pereira S, Silva J, Saboya C, Ramalho A (2013) Vitamin A Deficiency in Pregnancy: Perspectives after Bariatric Surgery. *Obesity Surgery*, **23**:249-254.

Chassaing B, Koren O, Goodrich J, Poole A, Srinivasan S, Ley R, Gewirtz A (2015) Dietary emulsifiers impact the mouse gut microbiota promoting colitis and metabolic syndrome *Nature* **519**, 92–96.

Chao MC, Hu SL, Hsu HS, Davidson L, Lin CH, Li CI, Liu CS, Li TC, Lin CC, Lin WY (2014) Serum homocysteine level is positively associated with chronic kidney disease in a Taiwan Chinese population. *Journal of Nephrology*, 2014.

Chaput J, Klingenberg L, Astrup A, Sjödin A (2011) Modern sedentary activities promote overconsumption of food in our current obesogenic environment. *Obesity Reviews*, **12**:5:e12–e20.

Chaput JP, Klingenberg L, Sjodin A (2010) Do all sedentary activities lead to weight gain: sleep does not. *Current opinion in clinical nutrition and metabolic care*, **13**(6):601-7.

Chavarro J. E., Toth T. L., Wright D. L., Meeker J. D., Hauser R. (2009) Body mass index in relation to semen quality, sperm DNA integrity, and serum reproductive hormone levels among men attending an infertility clinic. *Fertility and Sterility*, doi:10.1016/j.fertnstert.2009.01.100.

Chevallier JM (2010) Gastric banding using adjustable silastic ring in 2010. Technique, indications, results and management. *Journal of Visceral Surgery*, **147**: (5) e21-e29.

Chilelli N, Burlina S, Dalfrà MG, Lapolla A (2014) A Focus on the Impact of Bariatric Surgery on Pregnancy Outcome: Effectiveness, Safety and Clinical Management. *Journal of Obesity and Weight Loss Therapy*, **4**:210.

Chin J, Swamy G, Østbye T, Bastian L (2009) Contraceptive use by obese women 1 year postpartum. *Contraception*, **80**:5:463-8.

Chuang CH1, Chase GA, Bensyl DM, Weisman CS (2005) Contraceptive use by diabetic and obese women. *Womens Health Issues*, **15** (4):167-73.

Clemente J, Ursell L, Parfrey L, Knight R (2012) The Impact of the Gut Microbiota on Human Health: An Integrative View. *Cell*, **148**:6:1258–1270.

Clements R, Katasani V, Palepu R, Leeth R, Leath T, Roy B, Vickers S (2006) Incidence of vitamin deficiency after laparoscopic Roux-en-Y gastric bypass in a university hospital setting. *American Journal of Surgery*, **72**: 1196–1204.

Conterno L, Fava F, Viola R, Tuohy K (2011) Obesity and the gut microbiota: does up-regulating colonic fermentation protect against obesity and metabolic disease? *Genes & Nutrition*, **6**:3, 241-260.

Cornthwaite K, Jefferys A, Lenguerrand E, Hyde J, Lynch M, Draycott T, Johnson A, Siassakos D (2015) One size does not fit all. Management of the laparoscopic adjustable gastric band in pregnancy: a national prospective cohort study. *Lancet* **385**: S32.

Coupaye M, Puchaux K, Bogard C, Msika S, Jouet P, Clerici C, Larger E, Ledoux S (2009) Nutritional Consequences of Adjustable Gastric Banding and Gastric Bypass: A 1-year Prospective Study. *Obesity Surgery*, **19**:1:56-65.

Craig W & Mangels A (2009) American Dietetic Association Position of the American Dietetic Association: vegetarian diets. *Journal of the American Dietetic Association* **109**:7:1266-1282.

Crouter S, DellaValle D, Haas J (2013) Relationship between physical activity, physical performance, and iron status in adult women. *Applied Physiology Nutrition and Metabolism*, **37**:4:697-705.

Delzenne N, Neyrinck A, Bäckhed F, Cani P (2011) Targeting gut microbiota in obesity: effects of prebiotics and probiotics. *Nature Reviews Endocrinology*, **7**: 639-646.

Delzene N, Neyrinck A, Bäckhed F, Cani P (2011) Modulation of the gut microbiota by nutrients with prebiotic properties: consequences for host health in the context of obesity and metabolic syndrome. Microbial Cell Factories. Suppl.1:S10.

Devaraj S, Hemarajata P, Versalovic J (2013) The Human Gut Microbiome and Body Metabolism: Implications for Obesity and Diabetes. *Clinical Chemistry*, **59**: 4: 617-628.

Dhurander & Keith (2014) The aetiology of obesity beyond eating more and exercising less. *Best Practice and Research Clinical Gastroenterology* **28**:533-544.

DiBaise J, Frank D, Mathur R (2012) Impact of the Gut Microbiota on the Development of Obesity: Current Concepts. *American Journal of Gastroenterology Supplements* **1**:22-27.

di Frega AS, Dale B, Di Matteo L, Wilding M (2005) Secondary male factor infertility after Roux-en-Y gastric bypass for morbid obesity: case report. *Human Reproduction.* **20**: 997–998.

Dimitrios J. Pournaras and Carel W. le Roux (2009) After bariatric surgery, what vitamins should be measured and what supplements should be given? *Clinical Endocrinology,* **71**, 322–325 doi: 10.1111/j.1365-2265.2009.03564.x.

Dixon J, Dixon M, O-Brien P (2005) Birth Outcomes in Obese Women after Laparoscopic Adjustable Gastric Banding. *Obstetrics and Gynecology,* **106**:5:1.

Dixon J, Dixon M, O'Brien P (2001) Elevated homocysteine levels with weight loss after Lap-Band surgery: higher folate and vitamin B12 levels required to maintain homocysteine level. *International Journal of Obesity,* **25**: 219-227.

Ducarme G, Revaux A, Rodrigues A, Aissaoui F, Pharisien I, Uzan M (2007) Obstetric outcome following laparoscopic adjustable gastric banding. *International Journal of Gynaecology and Obstetrics,* **98**:3:244-7.

Du Plessis S, Cabler S, McAlister D, Sabanegh E, Agarwal A (2010) The effect of obesity on sperm disorders and male infertility. *Urology,* **7**:153- 161.

Efthymiou V, Hyphantis T, Karaivazoglou K, Gourzis P, Alexandrides TK, Kalfarentzos F, Assimakopoulos K (2014) The Effect of Bariatric Surgery on Patient HRQOL and Sexual Health During a 1-Year Postoperative Period. *Obesity surgery*. [Abstract only]. Available at: http://link.springer.com/article/10.1007/s11695-014-1384-x. Accessed 30th October 2014.

Eftekhari M, Mozaffari-Khosravi H, Shidfar F (2009) The relationship between BMI and iron status in iron-deficient adolescent Iranian girls. *Public Health Nutrition*, **12**(12):2377-81. doi: 10.1017/S1368980009005187. Epub 2009 Mar 12.

Enig M (1996) Health and Nutritional Benefits from Coconut Oil: An Important Functional Food for the 21st Century.

Ennemana A, Swartb K, Zillikensa M, van Dijka S, van Wijngaardenc J, Brouwer-Brolsmac E, Dhonukshe-Ruttenc R, Hofmana A, Rivadeneiraa F, van der Cammena T, Lipsd P, de Grootc C, Uitterlindena A, van Meursa J, van Schoorb N, van der Veldea N (2014) The association between plasma homocysteine levels and bone quality and bone mineral density parameters in older persons. *Bone*, **63**:141–146.

Ernst B, Thurnheer M, Schmid S, Schultes B (2009) Evidence for the Necessity to Systematically Assess Micronutrient Status Prior to Bariatric Surgery. *Obesity Surgery*, **19**:1:66-73.

Facchiano E, Iannell A, Santulli P, Mandelbrot L, Msika S (2012) Pregnancy after laparoscopic bariatric surgery: comparative study of adjustable gastric banding and Roux-en-Y gastric bypass. *Surgery for Obesity and Related Diseases* **8**:4:429–433

Flancbaum L, Belsley S, Drake V, Colarusso T, Tayler E (2006) Preoperative nutritional status of patients undergoing Roux-en-Y gastric bypass for morbid obesity. *Journal of Gastrointestinal Surgery,* **10**:7:1033-7.

Foodsafety.gov. U.S. Department of Health & Human Services. Available at: [http://www.foodsafety.gov /poisoning/risk/pregnant/chklist_pregnancy.html]. Accessed: 27th May 2014.

Foss Y (2009) Vitamin D deficiency is the cause of common obesity. *Medical Hypotheses,* **72**:3:314-21.

Fish E, Beverstein G, Olson D, Reinhardt S, Garren M, Gould J. (2010) Vitamin D Status of Morbidly Obese Bariatric Surgery Patients. *Journal of Surgical Research,* **164**: 198-202.

Freedhoff & Sharma (2010) Best Weight: A practical Guide to Office Based Obesity Management.

Freeth A, Prajuabpansri P, Victory J, Jenkins P (2012) Assessment of Selenium in Royx-en-Y Gastric Bypass and Gastric Banding Surgery. *Obesity Surgery,* **22**: 11: 1660-1665.

Furlani & Godoy (2008) Vitamins B1 and B2 contents in cultivated mushrooms. *Food Chemistry*, **106**:2:816–819.

Gadgil M, Chang H, Richards T, Gudzune K, Huizinga M, Clark J, Bennett W (2014) Laboratory testing for and diagnosis of nutritional deficiencies in pregnancy before and after bariatric surgery. *Journal of Womens Health* **23**:2:129-37.

Gaglarirmak (2011) Chemical Composition and Nutrition Value of Dried Cultivated Culinary-Medicinal Mushrooms from Turkey. *International Journal of Medicinal Mushrooms*, **13**:4:351-356.

García OP (2012) Effect of vitamin A deficiency on the immune response in obesity. *Proceedings of the Nutrition Society* **71**:2:290-7.

Gasteyger C, Suter M, Calmes JM, Gaillard RC, Giusti V. (2006) Changes in body composition, metabolic profile and nutritional status 24 months after gastric banding. *Obesity Surgery*, **16** (3): 243-250.

Georgia State University – Health Triangle PowerPoint. Available at: [http://wellness2.org/t/the-health-triangle-georgia-state-university-ppt-w37/]. Accessed: 20th November 2014.

Gesta S, Tseng Y, Kahn C (2007) Developmental origins of fat: tracking obesity to its source. *Cell*, **131**:2:242-256.

Gemmel K, Santry HP, Prachand VN, Alverdy JC (2009) Vitamin D deficiency in preoperative bariatric surgery patients. *Surgery for Obesity and Related Diseases*, **5**(1):54-9. doi: 10.1016/j.soard.2008.07.008. Epub 2008 Jul 24.

Gnacińska M, Małgorzewicz S, Stojek M, Łysiak-Szydłowska W, Sworczak K (2009) Role of Adipokines in complications related to obesity: A Review. *Advances in medical Science*, **54**:2:150-157.

González-Castejón M, Rodriguez-Casado A (2011) Dietary phytochemicals and their potential effects on obesity: A review. *Pharmacological Research* **64**:438–455.

Gosman G, King W, Schrope B, Steffen K, Strain G, Courcoulas A, Flum D, Pender J, Simhan H (2010) Reproductive Health of Women Electing Bariatric Surgery. *Fertility and Sterility*, **944**:1426–1431.

Gracia G, Altieri M, Pryor A (2014) OBGYN and Bariatric Surgery The Globesity Challenge to General Surgery pp 187-212.

Grant J (2012) Food for thought … and health. Making a case for plant-based nutrition. *Canadian Family Physician* **58**:9:917-919.

Greenberg J & Bell S (2011) Multivitamin Supplementation During Pregnancy: Emphasis on Folic Acid and l-Methylfolate. *Reviews in Obstetrics and Gynecology* **4**:3-4: 126–127.

Grimes C, Riddell L, Campbell K, Nowson C (2013) Dietary Salt Intake, Sugar-Sweetened Beverage Consumption, and Obesity Risk. *Pediatrics*, **101**:1:14 -21.

Grun F (2010) Obesogens. Current Opinions in Endocrinology Diabetes and Obesity. 17:5:453-9.

Guelinckx I, Devlieger R, Vansant G (2009) Reproductive outcome after bariatric surgery: a critical review. *Human Reproduction Update* **15**:2:189-201.

Hamalainen M, Nieminen R, Vuorela P, Heinonen M, Moilanen E (2007) Anti-Inflammatory Effects of Favonoids: Genistein, Kaempferol, Quercitin and Daidzein. *Mediators of Inflammation*: Article 45673.

Hammoud A, M. Gibson, S.C. Hunt, T.D. Adams, D.T. Carrell, R.L. Kolotkin, A.W. Meikle (2009) Effect of Roux-en-Y gastric bypass surgery on the sex steroids and quality of life in obese men. *Clinics in Endocrinology and Metabolism*, **94**:4:1329–1332.

Hannan, J. L., Maio, M. T., Komolova, M. & Adams, M. A. (2009) Beneficial impact of exercise and obesity interventions on erectile function and its risk factors. *Journal of Sexual Medicine,* **6** (Suppl. 3), 254–261.

Harris & Barger (2010) Specialised Care for Women Pregnant After Bariatric Surgery. *Journal of Midwifery & Women's Health*, **55**: 529-539.

Hezelgrave & Oteng-Ntim (2011) Pregancy after bariatric surgery: A review. *Journal of Obesity* Article ID 501939.

Hogeveen M, Blom H, Heijer M (2012) Maternal homocysteine and small-for-gestational-age offspring: systematic review and meta-analysis1,2 *American Journal of Clinical Nutrition*, **95**:1 130-136.

Hu F (2013) Resolved: there is sufficient scientific evidence that decreasing sugar-sweetened beverage consumption will reduce the prevalence of obesity and obesity-related diseases. *Obesity Reviews* **14**:8:606–619.

Hu F & Malik V (2010) Sugar-sweetened beverages and risk of obesity and type 2 diabetes: Epidemiologic evidence. *Physiology & Behavior*, **100**:1:47–54.

Haward R, Brown W, O'Brien P (2011) Does Pregnancy Increase the Need for Revisional Surgery After Laparoscopic Adjustable Gastric Banding? *Obesity Surgery*, **21**:9:1362-1369. [Abstract only].

Holick M & Chen T (2008) Vitamin D deficiency: a worldwide problem with health consequences. *American Journal of Clinical Nutrition*, **87**:4:1080S-6S.

Hu & Willett (2002) Optimal Diets for Prevention of Coronary Heart Disease *Journal of the American Medical Association* **288**:20:2569-2578.

Huber M, Knottnerus J, Green L, van der Horst H, Jadad A, Kromhout D, Leonard B, Lorig K, Loureiro M, van der Meer J, Schnabel P, Smith R, van Weel C, Smid H (2011) How should we define Health? *British Medical Journal*, **343**:d4163.

Hursel R, Viechtbauer W, Westerterp-Plantenga M (2009) The effects of green tea on weight loss and weight maintenance: a meta-analysis. *International Journal of Obesity* **33**, 956–961.

Hyman M (2007) Systems biology, toxins, obesity, and functional medicine. *Alternative Therapies in Health and Medicine* **13**:2:S134-S139.

Hyman M (2010) Environmental Toxins, Obesity and Diabetes: An Emerging Health Risk Factor. Alternative *Therapies in Health and Medicine* **16**:2:56-58.

Ignacio J (2013) Iron deficiency and bariatric surgery. *Nutrients* **5**:1595-1608.

Isidori A, Caprio M, Strollo F, Moretti C, Frajese G, Isidori A, Fabbri A (1999) Leptin and androgens in male obesity: evidence for leptin contribution to reduced androgen levels. *Journal of Clinical Endocrinology and Metabolism* **84**:3673–3680.

Isokangas P, Söderling E, Pienihäkkinen K, Alanen P (2000) Occurrence of Dental Decay in Children after Maternal Consumption of Xylitol Chewing Gum, a Follow-up from 0 to 5 Years of Age. *Journal of Dental Research,* **79**:11:1885-1889.

Jaiser & Winston (2010) Copper deficiency myelopathy. *Journal of Neurology* **257**:869-881.

Jefferys A, Siassakos D, Draycott T, Akande V, Fox R (2013) Deflation of gastric band balloon in pregnancy for improving outcomes. *Cochrane Database of Systematic Reviews*, **4**:CD010048.

Jiang Q (2014) Natural forms of vitamin E: metabolism, antioxidant, and anti-inflammatory activities and their role in disease prevention and therapy. *Free Radical Biology and Medicine*, **72**:76–90.

Jungheim E*, Travieso J, Hopeman M (2013) Weighing the impact of obesity on female reproductive function and fertility. *Nutrition Reviews*, **71**:S1:S3–S8.

Jurgens T & Whelan A (2014) Can green tea preparations help with weight loss? *Canadian Pharmacists Journal / Revue des Pharmaciens du Canada* **1715163514528668**.

Jurgens T, Whelan A, Killian L, Doucette S, Kirk S, Foy E. (2012) Green tea for weight loss and weight maintenance in overweight or obese adults. *Cochrane Database of Systematic Reviews*, **12**: CD008650.

Kane M, Pinkey J, Aasheim E, Barth J, Batterham R, Wellbourne R (2014) BOMSS Guidelines on perioperative and postoperative biochemical monitoring and micronutrient replacement for patients undergoing bariatric surgery. Available at: [http://www.bomss.org.uk /wp-content/uploads/2014/09/BOMSS-guidelines-Final-version1Oct14.pdf]. Accessed: 7th December 2014.

Kang J, Kondo F, Katayama Y (2006) Human exposure to bisphenol A. *Toxicology* **226**:2-3:79-89.

Katz (2008) *Nutrition in Clinical Practice 2nd Edn.*. Lippincott, Williiams & Wilkins. Philadelphia.

Katz D & Meller S (2014) Can We Say What Diet Is Best for Health? *Annual Review of Public Health* **35**: 83-103.

Kaska L, Kobiela J, Abacjew-Chmylko A, Chmylko L, Wojanowska-Pindel M, Kobiela P, Walerzak A, Makarewicz W, Proczko-Markuszewska M, Stefaniak T (2013) Nutrition and Pregnancy after Bariatric Surgery. International Scholarly Research Notices Obesity. Volume 2013: Article ID 492060.

Kasturi S. S., Tannir, J. & Brannigan R. E. (2008) The metabolic syndrome and male infertility. *Journal of Andrology,* **29**: 251–259.

Khan R, Dawlatly B, Chappatte O (2013) Pregnancy outcome following bariatric surgery. *The Obstetrician & Gynaecologist,* **15**:37–43.

Kim & Kim (2011) Effect of garlic on high fat induced obesity. *Acta Biologica Hungaria.* **62**:3:244-254.

Kimata H (2010) Modulation of fecal polyamines by viewing humorous films in patients with atopic dermatitis. *European Journal of Gastroenterology and Hepatology,* **22**:6:724-8.

Kjær MM, Lauenborg J, Breum BM, MD, Nilas L (2013) The risk of adverse pregnancy outcome after bariatric surgery: a nationwide register-based matched cohort study. *American Journal of Obstetrics and Gynecology* **208**:6:464.e1–464.e5.

Kominiarek (2011) Preparing for and managing a pregnancy after bariatric surgery. *Seminars in Perinatology* **35**:6:356–361.

Konttinen H, Männistöb S, Sarlio-Lähteenkorvac S, Silventoinend K, Haukkalaa A (2010) Emotional eating, depressive symptoms and self-reported food consumption. A population-based study. *Appetite* **54**:3:473–479.

Kulick D, Hark L, Deen D (2010) Bariatric Surgery Patient: A growing Role for Registered Dieticians. *Journal of the American Dietetic Association*, **110** (4): 593-599.

Kumar D, Kumar S, Singh J, Rashmi N, Vashistha B, Singh N (2010) Free Radical Scavenging and Analgesic Activities of Cucumis sativus L. Fruit Extract. *Journal of Young Pharmacists* 2:4: 365–368.

Lanthier & Leclercq (2014) Adipose tissue as endocrine target organs. *Best Practice & Research Clinical Gastroenterology* **28:**545-558.

Lapolla A, Marangon M, Dalfrà MG, Segato G, De Luca M, Fedele D, Favretti F, Enzi G, Busetto L. (2010) Pregnancy outcome in morbidly obese women before and after laparoscopic gastric banding. *Obesity Surgery* **20**:9:1251-7.

Lazaros L, Hatzi E, Markoula S, Takenaka A, Sofikitis N, Zikopoulos K, I. Georgiou I (2012) Dramatic reduction in sperm parameters following bariatric surgery: report of two cases. *Andrologia* **44**:428–432.

Lecube A, Zafon C, Gromaz A, Fort J, Caubet E, Baena J, Tortosa F (2015) Iodine deficiency is higher in morbid obesity in comparison with late after bariatric surgery and non-obese women. *Obesity Surgery*. 25:1:85-9.

Lee P, Smith S, Linderman J, Courville A, Brychta R, Dieckmann W, Werner C, Chen K, Celi F (2014) Temperature-acclimated brown adipose tissue modulates insulin sensitivity in humans Published online before print June 22, 2014, doi: 10.2337/db14-0513. *Diabetes*. [Abstract only].

Legro R, Kunselman A, Meadows J, Kesner J, Krieg E, Rogers A, Cooney R (2014) Time-related increase in urinary testosterone levels and stable semen analysis parameters after bariatric surgery in men. *Reproductive BioMedicine Online*. In Press, Uncorrected Proof. Available at: [http://www.sciencedirect.com]. Accessed: 20th November 2014.

Lesser L, Ebbeling C, Goozner M, Wypij D, Ludwig D (2007) Relationship between funding source and conclusion among nutrition-related scientific articles. *PLoS Medicine* **4**:1:e5.

Ley R (2010) Obesity and the human micro-biome. *Current Opinion in Gastroenterology* **26**:5-11.

Li K, Kaaks R, Linseisen J, Rohrmann S (2012) Associations of dietary calcium intake and calcium supplementation with myocardial infarction and stroke risk and overall cardiovascular mortality in the Heidelberg cohort of the European Prospective Investigation into Cancer and Nutrition study (EPIC-Heidelberg). *Heart*, **98**: 920-925.

Liau Kai Ming, Lee Yeong Yeh, Chen Chee Keong, Rasool Aida Hanum (2011) An Open-Label Pilot Study to Assess the Efficacy and Safety of Virgin Coconut Oil in Reducing Visceral Adiposity. *Pharmacology* **949686**.

Lima K, Lima R, Gonçalves M, Faintuch J, Morais L, Asciutti L, Costa M (2014) High Frequency of Serum Chromium Deficiency and Association of Chromium with Triglyceride and Cholesterol Concentrations in Patients Awaiting Bariatric Surgery. *Obesity Surgery* **24**:771–776.

Limaye & Salvi (2014) Obesity and Asthma: The Role of Environmental Pollutants. *Immunology and Allergy Clinics of North America* **34**:4:839–855.

Linus Pauling Institute at Oregon State University. Available at: [http://lpi.oregonstate.edu/infocenter /minerals/iron/#]. Accessed: 20th May 2012.

Linus Pauling Institute at Oregon State University. Pregnancy and Lactation. Available at: [http://lpi.oregonstate.edu/infocenter/lifestages/pregnanc yandlactation/]. Accessed: 10th May 2013.

Liu (2003) Health benefits of fruit and vegetables are from additive and synergistic combinations of phytochemicals. *American Journal of Clinical Nutrition* **78**:3:517S-520S.

Lo Menzo E, Cappellani A, Zanghi A, Di Vita M, Berretta M, Szomstein S (2014) Nutritional Implications of Obesity: Before and After Bariatric Surgery. *Bariatric Surgical Practice and Patient Care* **9**: 1.

Louie J, Flood V, Hector D, Rangan A, Gill T (2011) Dairy consumption and overweight and obesity: a systematic review of prospective cohort studies.

Obesity Reviews **12**:7:e582–e592.

Ludwig & Willett (2013) Three Daily Servings of Reduced-Fat Milk An Evidence-Based Recommendation? *JAMA Pediatrics* **167**:9:788-789.

Luppino F, de Wit L, Bouvy P, Stijnen T, Cuijpers P, Penninx B, Zitman F (2010) Overweight, obesity and depression. *General Archives of Psychiatry* **63**:3:220-229.

Lynch B (2014) MTHFR Made Easy.
[http://www.blogtalkradio.com/undergroundwellness/2014/11/19/dr-ben-lynch-mthfr-made-easy]. Accessed: 30th November 2014.

Maggard M, Yermilov I, Li Z, Maglione M, Newberry S, Suttorp M, Hilton L, Santry HP, Morton JM, Livingston EH, Shekelle PG (2008) Pregnancy and fertility following bariatric surgery: a systematic review. *JAMA* **300**:19:2286-96.

Maggard-Gibbons M (2014) Optimizing Micronutrients in Pregnancies Following Bariatric Surgery. *Journal of Women's Health* **23**:2: 107-107.

Maggard M, Li Z, Yermilov I, Maglione M, Suttorp M, Carter J, Tringale C, Hilton L, Chen S, Shekelle P. Bariatric Surgery in Women of Reproductive Age: Special Concerns for Pregnancy. Evidence Report/Technology Assessment No. 169. (Prepared by the Southern California Evidence-based Practice Center under Contract No. 290-02-003). Rockville, MD: Agency for Healthcare Research and Quality. November 2008. Available from: http://www.ncbi.nlm.nih.gov/books/NBK38559/.

Malik V, Popkin B, Bray G, Després JP, Hu F (2010) Sugar-Sweetened Beverages, Obesity, Type 2 Diabetes Mellitus, and Cardiovascular Disease Risk. *Circulation* **121**: 1356-1364.

Malik V, Pan A, Willett W, Hu F (2013) Sugar-sweetened beverages and weight gain in children and adults: a systematic review and meta-analysis. *AJCN* **98**:4:1084-1102.

Manichanh C, Eck A, Varela E, Roca J, Clemente J, González A, Knights D, Knight R, Estrella S, Hernandez C, Guyonnet D, Accarino A, Santos J, Malagelada J, Guarner F, Azpiroz F (2014) Anal gas evacuation and colonic microbiota in patients with flatulence: effect of diet. *Gut* **63**:401-408.

Manning P, Sutherland W, Walker R, Williams S, deJong S, Ryalls A, Berry E (2004) Effect of High-Dose Vitamin E on Insulin Resistance and Associated Parameters in Overweight Subjects. *Diabetes Care* **27**:9:2166-2171.

Martineau & Khan (2014) Maternal Vitamin D insufficiency is associated with adverse pregnancy and neonatal outcomes. *Evidence Based Medicine* 2014;**19**:e4 doi:10.1136/eb-2013-101368 [Abstract only].

Mastromarino P, Vitali B, Mosca L (2013) Bacterial vaginosis: a review on clinical trials with probiotics. *New MicrobIological* **36**, 229-238.

Mechanick J, Kushner R, Sugerman H, Gonzalez-Campoy J, Collazo-Clavell M, Spitz A, Apovian C, Livingston E, Brolin R, Sarwer D, Anderson W, Dixon J (2009) American Association of Clinical Endocrinologists, The Obesity Society, and American Society for Metabolic & Bariatric Surgery Medical Guidelines for Clinical Practice for the Perioperative Nutritional, Metabolic, and Non-surgeical Support of the Bariatric Surgery Patient. Available at: http://www.sunut.org.uy/wp-content/uploads/2012/11/guias-AACE-TOS-ASMBS-BARIATRICA.pdf. Accessed: 20th March 2012.

Mechanick J, Youdim A, Jones, D, Garvey T, Hurley D, McMahon M, Heinberg L, Kushner R, Adams T, Shikora S, Dixon J, Brethauer S (2013) Clinical Practice Guidelines for the Perioperative Nutritional, Metabolic, and Nonsurgical Support of the Bariatric Surgery Patient -2013 Update: Cosponsored by American Association of Clinical Endocrinologists, The Obesity Society, and American Society for Metabolic & Bariatric Surgery. AACE/TOS/ASMBS Guidelines. *Surgery for Obesity and Related Disease* **9**:159-191.

Matteis R, Lucertinia F, Guescinia M, Polidoria E, Zeppaa S, Stocchia V, Cintib S, Cuppinic R (2013) Exercise as a new physiological stimulus for brown adipose tissue activity. *Nutrition, Metabolism and Cardiovascular Diseases* **23**:6:582–590.

McCance and Widdowson's The Composition of Foods, Sixth Summary Edition. Foods Standards Agency (2004) Cambridge Royal Society of Chemistry. London.

McClung & Karl (2009) Iron deficiency and obesity: the contribution of inflammation and diminished iron absorption. *Nutrition Reviews* **67**:2:100-4.

Medeiros M, Saunders C, Chagas C, Pereira S, Saboya C, Ramalho A (2013) Vitamin D deficiency in Pregnancy after Bariatric Surgery. *Obesity Surgery* **23**:1679-1684.

Meier U & Gressner A (2004) Endocrine Regulation of Energy Metabolism: Review of Pathobiochemical and Clinical Chemical Aspects of Leptin, Ghrelin, Adiponectin, and Resistin. *Clinical Chemistry* **50**:9:1511-1525

Missouri Bariatric Services: Guidelines Before and After Bariatric Surgery. Available at: [http://www.muhealth.org /services/surgical/bariatrics/]. Accessed 20th February 2012.

Mitchell & de Zwaan (2011) Psychosocial Assessment and Treatment of Bariatric Surgery Patients. Cummings and Furtado, Chapter 9 Nutritional Care of the Bariatric Surgery Patient p.159. Taylor and Francis Group, USA.

Miyashita K (2009) The carotenoid fucoxanthin from brown seaweed affects obesity. *Lipid Technology* **21**:8-9:186–190.

Mohamed S, Hashim S, Rahman H (2012) Seaweeds: A sustainable functional food for complementary and alternative therapy. *Trends in Food Science & Technology* **23**:2:83–96.

Moroshko I, Brennan L, Warren N, Brown W, O'Brien P (2014) Patients' Perspectives on Laparoscopic Adjustable Gastric Banding (LAGB) Aftercare Attendance: Qualitative Assessment. *Obesity Surgery* **24**:2:266-275.

Morton G, Meek T, Schwartz M (2014) Neurobiology of food intake in health and disease. *Nature Reviews Neuroscience* **15**:367–378.

Mozaffari-Khosravi H, Ahadi Z & Tafti M, (2014) The Effect of Green Tea versus Sour Tea on Insulin Resistance, Lipids Profiles and Oxidative Stress in Patients with Type 2 Diabetes Mellitus: A Randomized Clinical Trial. *Iranian Journal of Medical Science* **39**:5: 424–432.

Mullin G & Delzenne (2014) The Human Gut Microbiome and Its Role in Obesity and the Metabolic Syndrome Integrative Weight Management. *Nutrition and Health* 2014, pp 71-105.

Mutzel M (2014) How to Turn your Gut Bacteria into Fat Burning Machines: [http://www.blogtalkradio.com /undergroundwellness/2014/11/19/mike-mutzel].

Natural Standard: The Authority on Integrative Medicine Available at: [http://naturalstandard.com] Accessed: 30th November 2014.

Nakamura K, Haglind E, Clowes J, Achenbach S, Atkinson E, Melton L, Kennel K (2014) Fracture risk following bariatric surgery: a population-based study. *Osteoporosis International* **25**:1:151-158. Abstract only.

Niu X, Chen X, Xiao Y, Dong J, Zhang R, Lu M, Kong W (2014) The Differences in Homocysteine Level between Obstructive Sleep Apnea Patients and Controls: A Meta-Analysis. *PLoS ONE* **9**:4: e95794.

Nutter S (2003) *The Health Triangle*. Anchor Points Inc. USA.

Odegaard J, Chawla A (2012) Connecting type 1 and type 2 diabetes through innate immunity. *Cold Spring Harbour Perspectives in Medicine* **2**:3:a007724.

Office of Dietary Supplements (2013) Available at: [http://ods.od.nih.gov/factsheets].

O'Kane M, Pinkney J, Aasheim E, Barth J, Batterham R, Welbourn R (2014) BOMSS Guidelines on peri-operative and postoperative biochemical monitoring and micronutrient replacement for patients undergoing bariatric surgery. Available at: [http://www.bomss.org.uk /wp-content/uploads/2014/09/BOMSS-guidelines-Final-version1Oct14.pdf].

Onakpoya I, Spencer E, Heneghana C, Thompson M (2014) The effect of green tea on blood pressure and lipid profile: A systematic review and meta-analysis of randomized clinical trials. *Nutrition, Metabolism and Cardiovascular Diseases* **24**:8:823–836.

Oster E (2013) *Expecting Better.* Orion Publishing Group Limited.

Ostlund M, Backman O, Marsk R, Stockeld D, Lagergren J, Rasmussen F, Näslund E (2013) Increased admission for alcohol dependence after gastric bypass surgery compared with restrictive bariatric surgery. *JAMA Surgery* **148**:4:374-7.

Ota K, Dambaeva S, Han AR, Beaman K, Gilman-Sachs A, Kwak-Kim J (2014) Vitamin D deficiency may be a risk factor for recurrent pregnancy losses by increasing cellular immunity and autoimmunity. *Human Reproduction* **29**:2: 208-219.

Palmer N, Bakos H, Fullston T, Lane M (2012) Impact of obesity on male fertility, sperm function and molecular composition. *Spermatogenesis* **2**:4: 253–263.

Patel S & Hu F (2008) Short Sleep Duration and Weight Gain: A Systematic Review. *Obesity* **16**:3:643–653.

Papadopouloua E, Vafeiadia M, Agramuntf S, Mathianakig K, Karakostag P, Spanakih A, Besselinki H, Kivirantaj H, Rantakokkoj P, Sarrig K, Koutisg A, Chatzig L, Kogevinas M (2013) Maternal diet, prenatal exposure to dioxins and other persistent organic pollutants and anogenital distance in children. *Science of The Total Environment 461-462:222–229.*

Pearce S, Cheetham T (2010) Diagnosis and management of vitamin D deficiency. *British Medical Journal* **340**:b5664.

Pennington & Spungen (2010) *Bowes and Church's Food Values of Portions Commonly used. 19th Edn.* Lippincott, Williams and Wilkins, Philadelphia.

Peirce V, Carobbio S, Vidal-Puig A (2014) The different shades of fat. *Nature* **510**, 76–83.

Pestana D, Faria G, Sá C, Fernandes V, Teixeira D, Norberto S, Faria A, Meireles M, Marques C, Correia-Sá L, Cunha A, Guimarães J, Taveira-Gomes A, Santos A, Domingues V, Delerue-Matos C, Monteiro R, Calhau C (2014) Persistent organic pollutant levels in human visceral and subcutaneous adipose tissue in obese individuals-- depot differences and dysmetabolism implications. *Environironmental Research* **133**:170-7.

Pilone V, Ariola Hasani, Rosa Di Micco, Antonio Vitiello, Angela Monda, Giuliano Izzo, Leucio Iacobelli, Elisabetta Villamaina, Pietro Forestieri (2014) Pregnancy after laparoscopic gastric banding: Maternal and neonatal outcomes. *International Journal of Surgery* **12**: S1:S136–S139.

Pinhas-Hamiel O, Newfield R, Koren I, Agmon A, Lilos P, Phillip M (2003) Greater prevalence of iron deficiency in overweight and obese children and adolescents. *International Journal of Obesity Related Metabolic Disorders* **27**:3:416-8.

Poddar K, Ames M, Hsin-Jen C, Feeney MJ, Wang Y, Cheskin L (2013) Positive effect of mushrooms substituted for meat on body weight, body composition, and health parameters. A 1-year randomized clinical trial. *Appetite* **71**:379-87.

Powell (2013) *Medicinal Mushrooms: The Essential Guide.* Mycology Press.

Prentice A (2003) Thin babies with excess body fat may explain later adiposity in Indians Intrauterine factors, adiposity, and hyperinsulinaemia. *British Medical Journal* **327**:7420: 880–881.

Rajapakse & Kim (2011) *Chapter 2: Nutritional and Digestive Health Benefits of Seaweed.* Marine Medicinal Foods: Implications and Applications, Macro and Microalgae. Academic Press. pp.17-27 Available at: [http://books.google.co.uk/books]. Accessed: 20th November 2014.

Randolph T (1947) Masked food allergy as a factor in the development and persistence of obesity. Proceedings of the Annual Meeting. *Central Society for Clinical Research (U S)*. **1947**:20:85.

Rayalam S, Della-Fera M, Baile C (2008) Phytochemicals and regulation of the adipocyte life cycle. *Journal of Nutritional Biochemistry* **19**:717-726.

Ready & Burton (2011) *Neuro-linguistic Programming For Dummies*. John Wiley & Sons Ltd. West Sussex.

Reid I (2002) Relationships among body mass, its components, and bone. Bone. 2002 Nov;31(5):547-55.

Reis L & Dias F (2012) Male Fertility, Obesity, and Bariatric Surgery. *Reproductive Sciences* **19**:8:778-785.

Reis L, Zani E, Saad R, Chaim E, de Oliveira L, Fregonesi A (2012) Bariatric Surgery Does not Interfere With Sperm Quality—A Preliminary Long-Term Study. *Reproductive Sciences* **19**:10 1057-1062.

Riess K, Farnen J, Lambert P, Mathiason M, Kothari S (2009) Ascorbic acid deficiency in bariatric surgical population. *Surgery for Obesity and Related Diseases* **5**:1:81-6.

Rop O, Mlcek J, Jurikova T (2009) Beta-glucans in higher fungi and their health effects. *Nutrition Reviews* **67**:11:624–631.

Rosen & Spiegelman (2014) What we talk about when we talk about fat. *Cell* **156**:20-44.

Rudel R, Gray J, Engel C,Rawsthorne T, Dodson R, Ackerman J, Rizzo J, Nudelman J, Brody J (2011) . Food packaging and bisphenol A and Bis (2-ethylhexyl) phthalate exposure: findings from a dietary intervention. *Environmental Health Perspec*tives **119**:914-920.

Sadiqulla M, Khan I, Rahmath A (2014) Serum homocysteine as a risk factor in diabetic with colour vision deficiency and for developing retinopathy. *International Journal of Science and Public Health* **3**:2:165-168.

Safer D, Adler S, Robinson A, Darcy A, Cook C (2013) Factors Distinguishing Weight-Loss Success and Failure at 5 or More Years Post Bariatric Surgery. Stanford School of Medicine & Bariatric Support Centre International.

Sala-Vila A & Ramon Estruch & Emilio Ros (2015) New Insights into the Role of Nutrition in CVD Prevention. *Current Cardiology Reports* **17:26**.

Sanchez M, Darimont C, Drapeau V, Emady-Azar S, Lepage M, Rezzonico E, Ngom-Bru C, Berger B, Philippe L, Ammon-Zuffrey C, Leone P, Chevrier G, St-Amand E, Marette A, Doré J, Tremblay A (2014). Effect of Lactobacillus rhamnosus CGMCC1.3724 supplementation on weight loss and maintenance in obese men and women. *British Journal of Nutrition* **111**:1507-1519.

Sanz Y, Rastmanesh R, Agostonic C (2013) Understanding the role of gut microbes and probiotics in obesity: How far are we? *Pharmacological Research* **69**:1:144–155.

Sarwer D, Sptizer J, Wadden T, Mitchell J, Lancaster K, Courcoulas A, Gourash W, Rosen R, Christian N (2014) Changes in sexual functioning and sex hormone levels in women following bariatric surgery. *JAMA Surgery* **149**:1: 26–33.

Schweiger C, Weiss R, Berry E, Keidar A (2010) Nutritional Deficiencies in Bariatric Surgery Candidates. *Obesity Surgery* **20:2**:193-197.

Sermondade N, Massinc N, Boitrelled F, Pfeffere J, Eustachea F, Sifera C, Czernichowf S, Lévya R (2012) Sperm parameters and male fertility after bariatric surgery: three case series. *Reproductive BioMedicine Online* **24**:2:206–210.

Shankar P, Boylan M, Sriram K (2010) Micronutrient deficiencies after bariatric surgery. *Nutrition* **26**:11–12:1031–1037.

Shahrook S, Hanada N, Sawada K, Ota E, Mori R (2014) Vitamin K supplementation during pregnancy for improving outcomes (Protocol) *The Cochrane Library* CD010920.

Sharpe R & Drake A (2013) Obesogens and obesity—An alternative view? *Obesity* **21**:6:1081–1083.

Sheiner E, Willis K, Yogev Y (2013) Bariatric Surgery: Impact on Pregnancy Outcomes. *Current Diabetes Reports* **13**:1:19-26.

Shen J, Obin M, Zhao L (2013) The gut microbiota, obesity and insulin resistance. *Molecular Aspects of Medicine* **34**:1:39–58.

Singh & Kumar (2007) Wernicke encephalopathy after obesity surgery: A systematic review. *Neurology* **68**:11:807-811.

Skowrońska-Jóźwiak E, Adamczewski Z, Tyszkiewicz A, Krawczyk-Rusiecka K, Lewandowski K, Lewiński A (2014) Assessment of adequacy of vitamin D supplementation during pregnancy. *Annals of Agricultural and Environmental Medicine* **21**:1:198-200].

Skull A, Slater G, Duncombe J, Fielding G (2004) Laparoscopic adjustable banding in pregnancy: safety, patient tolerance and effect on obesity-related pregnancy outcomes. *Obesity Surgery* **14**:2:230-235.

Soleymani T, Tejavanija S, Morgan S (2011) Obesity, bariatric surgery, and bone. *Current Opinion in Rheumatology* **23**:4:396–405.

Stanhope K, Medici V, Bremer A, Lee V, Lam H, Nunez M, Chen G, Keim N, Havel P (2015) A dose-response study of consuming high-fructose corn syrup–sweetened beverages on lipid/lipoprotein risk factors for cardiovascular disease in young adults. American Journal of Clinical Nutrition **ajcn100461.**

Svensson P, Anveden A, Romeo S, Peltonen M, Ahlin S, Burza M, Carlsson B, Jacobson P, Lindroos AK, Lönroth H, Maglio C, Näslund I, Sjöholm K, Wedel H, Söderpalm B, Sjöström L, Carlsson L (2013) Alcohol consumption and alcohol problems after bariatric surgery in the Swedish obese subjects study. *Obesity* **21**:12:2444–2451.

Tchoukalova Y, Votruba S, Tchkonia T, Giorgadze N, Kirkland J, Jensen M (2010) Regional differences in cellular mechanisms of adipose tissue gain with overfeeding. *PNAS* **107**:18226-18231.

Thaiss C, Zeevi D, Levy M, Zilberman-Schapira G, Suez J, Tengeler A, Abramson L, Katz M, Korem T, Zmora N, Kuperman Y, Biton I, Gilad S, Harmelin A, Shapiro H, Halpern Z, Segal E, Elinav E (2014) Transkingdom Control of Microbiota Diurnal Oscillations Promotes Metabolic Homeostasis *Cell.* **159**:3:514–529.

The Physicians Committee for Responsible Medicine (2014) Available at: [http://www.pcrm.org/health /diets/vegdiets/health-concerns-about-dairy-products]. Accessed: 4th December 2014.

Traber MG. Vitamin E. In: Shils ME, Shike M, Ross AC, Caballero B, Cousins R, eds. (2006) Modern Nutrition in Health and Disease. 10th ed. Baltimore, MD: Lippincott Williams & Wilkins 396-411.

Tsai CW, Chen HW, Sheenb LY, Liia CK (2012) Garlic: Health benefits and actions. *BioMedicine* **2**:1:17–29.

Tu CP, Yang HM, Lin KW, Akgül B, Chen YH, Lu TH, Hsieh L, Ching YH, Chen CH, Kikuchi T, Chen YT (2011) Dietary garlic prevents development of or alleviates diabetes and obesity in mice. *The FASEB Journal* **25**:204.2.

Turner-McGrievy G, Davidson C, Wingard E, Wilcox S, Frongillo E, (2015) Comparative effectiveness of plant-based diets for weight loss: A randomized controlled trial of five different diets. *Nutrition.* **31**:2:350–358.

Van Cauter E, Knutson K (2008) Sleep and the epidemic of obesity in children and adults. *European Journal of Endocrinology*, **159**: S59-S66.

Van Mieghem T, Van Schoubroeck D, Depiere M, Debeer A, Hanssens M (2008) Fetal cerebral hemorrhage caused by vitamin K deficiency after complicated bariatric surgery. *Obstetrics and Gynecology* **112**:2:2:434-6.

Veyrune J, Miller C, Czernichow S, Ciangura C, Nicolas E, Hennequin M (2008) Impact of Morbid Obesity on Chewing Ability. *Obesity Surgery* **18**:11:1467-1472.

Vicennati V, Garelli S, Rinaldi E , Dalmazi G, Pagotto U, Pasquali R (2014) Cross-talk between adipose tissue and the HPA axis in obesity and overt hypercortisolemic states. *Hormone Molecular Biology and Clinical Investigation* **17**:2:63–77. Abstract only.

Villarroya F & Vidal-Puig A (2013) Beyond the Sympathetic Tone: The New Brown Fat Activators. *Cell Metabolism* **17**:5:638–643.

Vitamin A and Carotenoids - Office of Dietary Supplements National Institute of Health [http://ods.od.nih.gov]. Accessed: May 2012.

Von Mach M-A, Stoeckli R, Bilz S, Kraenzlin M, Langer I, Keller U (2004) Changes in bone mineral content after surgical treatment of morbid obesity. *Metabolism*, **53** (7): 918-921.

Vrebosch L, Bel S, Vansant G, Guelinckx I, Devlieger R (2012) Maternal and neonatal outcome after laparoscopic adjustable gastric banding: a systematic review. *Obesity Surgery* **22**:10:1568-79.

Wang & Beydoun (2007) The Obesity Epidemic in the United States – Gender, Age, Socio-economic, Racial/Ethnic, and Geographic Characteristics. *Epidemiologic Reviews*, **29**:1: 6-28.

Watson & Preedy (2012) *Bioactive Food as Dietary Interventions for Diabetes: Bioactive Foods in Chronic Disease States.* Elsevier. Academic Press.

Williams D, Edwards D, Hamernig I, Jian L, James A, Johnson S, Tapsell L (2013) Vegetables containing phytochemicals with potential anti-obesity properties: A review. *Food Research International* **52**:1:323–333.

Williamson, (2006) Nutrition in Pregnancy. *Nutrition Bulletin* **31**:1:28–59.

Wilson (2014) MTHFR, CBS and COMT defects and Nutritional Balancing. The Centre For Development. Available at: [http://drlwilson.com/Articles /FOLIC%20ACID%20DEFECTS.htm]. Accessed: 2nd December 2014.

Wingard D, Berkman L, Brand R (1982) A Multivariate Analysis of Health-related Practices. A Nine-Year Mortality Follow-up of the Alameda County Study. *American Journal of Epidemiology* **116**:5: 765-775.

World Health Organisation Definition Of Health (1948) Available at: [http://www.who.int/about/definition/en /print.html]. Accessed: 30th November 2014.

World Health Organisation (2013) *Guideline: Calcium supplementation in pregnant women.* Available at: [http://apps.who.int/iris/bitstream/10665/85120/1/97892 41505376_eng.pdf?ua=1]. Accessed: 20th November 2014.

Wolf K & Lorenz R (2012) Gut Microbiota and Obesity. *Current Obesity Reports,* **1**:1-8.

Wortsman J, Matsuoka L, Chen T, Lu Z, Holick M (2003) Decreased bioavailability of vitamin D in obesity. *American Journal of Clinical Nutrition* **72**:3:690-3.

Wozniak S, Gee L, Wachtel M, Frezza E (2009) Adipose tissue : the new endocrine organ? A review article. *Digestive Diseases and Sciences* **54**:9:1847-1856.

Whalley L, Duthie S, Collins A, Starr J, Deary I, Lemmon H, Duthie A, Murray A, Staff R (2014) Homocysteine, antioxidant micronutrients and late onset dementia. *European Journal of Nutrition* **53**:1:277-285.

Xanthakos S (2009) Nutritional Deficiencies in Obesity and After Bariatric Surgery. *Pediatric Clinical North America* **56**:5: 1105–1121.

Yetley E (2008) Assessing the vitamin D status of the US population. *American Journal of Clinical Nutrition* **88**:2:558S-564S.

Yong J, Ge L, Ng YF, Tan SN (2009) The Chemical Composition and Biological Properties of Coconut (Cocos nucifera L.) Water. *Molecule* **14**:5144-5164.

Yong SB, Wua CC, Wangb L, Yang KD (2013) Influence and Mechanisms of Maternal and Infant Diets on the Development of Childhood Asthma. *Pediatrics & Neonatology* **54**:1:5–11.

Young (2007) How to increase serotonin in the human brain without drugs. *Journal of Psychiatry Neuroscience* **32**:6:394–399.

Index

A

Adjustments, 72, 100

Adipose tissue, 20, 22, 212, 231, 232, 237, 241, 247, 248, 250

Adrenal Stress Questionnaire, 44

Alkalising Juice, 154

American Association of Clinical Endocrinologists, 4, 236, 237

American Society for Metabolic and Bariatric Surgery, 4

Angry fat, 21, 23

Anti-inflammatory, xiii, 53, 87, 102, 104, 105, 106, 107, 109, 128, 149, 226, 229

Apple, almond and cinnamon pancakes, 177

Avocado Smoothie, 156

B

Band Fill, 93, 100

Band Loosened, xi, 76, 77

Band Mechanics, xi, 77

Beet It, 154

Beetroot Buzz, 158

Benefits, ix, 7, 8, 16, 85, 107, 108, 140, 222, 234, 242, 247

Berry Breakfast, 153

Berry Smoothie, 156

Biochemical Tests, xiv, 193, 195, 207

Bio-toxicity, x, 48

Bio-toxicity Symptom Questionnaire, 51-52

Blood sugar imbalance, 41, 82

Bone broth, 159

Bone Health, ix, 28

Breakfast, xiii, 98, 103, 185

Breakfasts, 81, 94, 97, 110, 148, 152, 153, 175

British Obesity and Metabolic Surgery Society, 4, 196

H

I

J

K

L

M

N

O

P

Q

R

S

W

Z

46056377R00151

Made in the USA
Charleston, SC
10 September 2015